THE BOSTON
FLOATING HOSPITAL

THE BOSTON
FLOATING HOSPITAL

How a BOSTON HARBOR BARGE
changed the course of PEDIATRIC MEDICINE

THE FIRST ONE HUNDRED YEARS

LUCIE PRINZ
with JACOBA VAN SCHAIK

Tufts Medical Center, Boston, MA
www.floatinghospital.org

Printed in U.S.A. First Edition © 2014

Library of Congress Cataloging-in-Publication Data

Prinz, Lucie, 1931-
   The Boston Floating Hospital : how a Boston harbor barge changed the course of pediatric medicine : the first one hundred years / Lucie Prinz ; with Jacoba Van Schaik.
      pages cm
   Includes bibliographical references and index.
   1. Boston Floating Hospital--History. 2. Boston Floating Hospital for Infants and Children--History. 3. Children--Hospitals--Massachusetts--Boston--History. 4. Hospital ships--Massachusetts--Boston--History. I. Van Schaik, Jacoba. II. Title.
   RJ28.B7P75 2014
   362.19892009744'61--dc23
                        2014023434
   ISBN HC: 978-1-934598-14-6
   ISBN PB: 978-1-934598-15-3

Book and cover design by Holly Gordon. www.missgordon.com

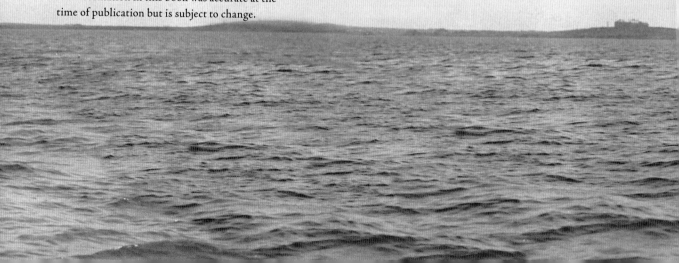

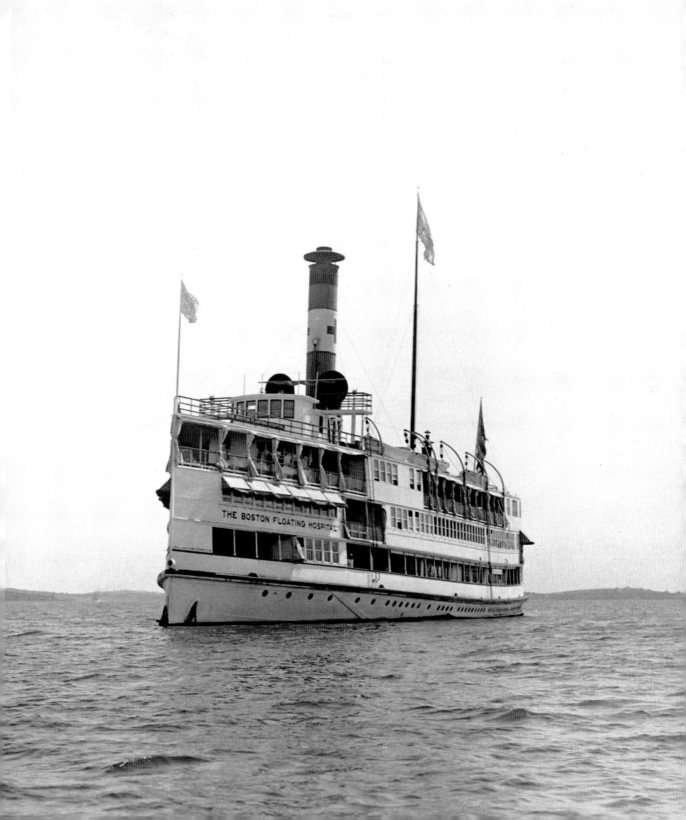

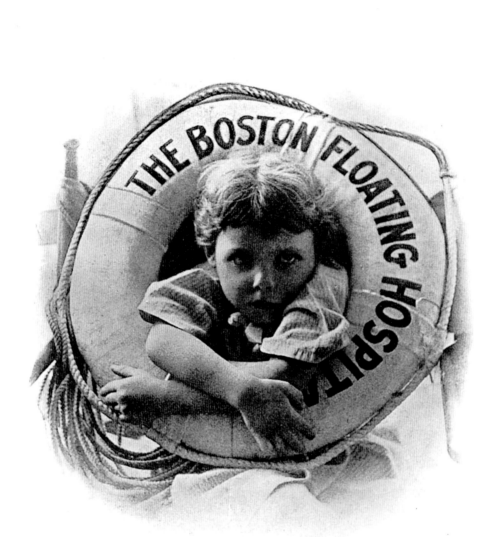

TABLE *of* CONTENTS

—

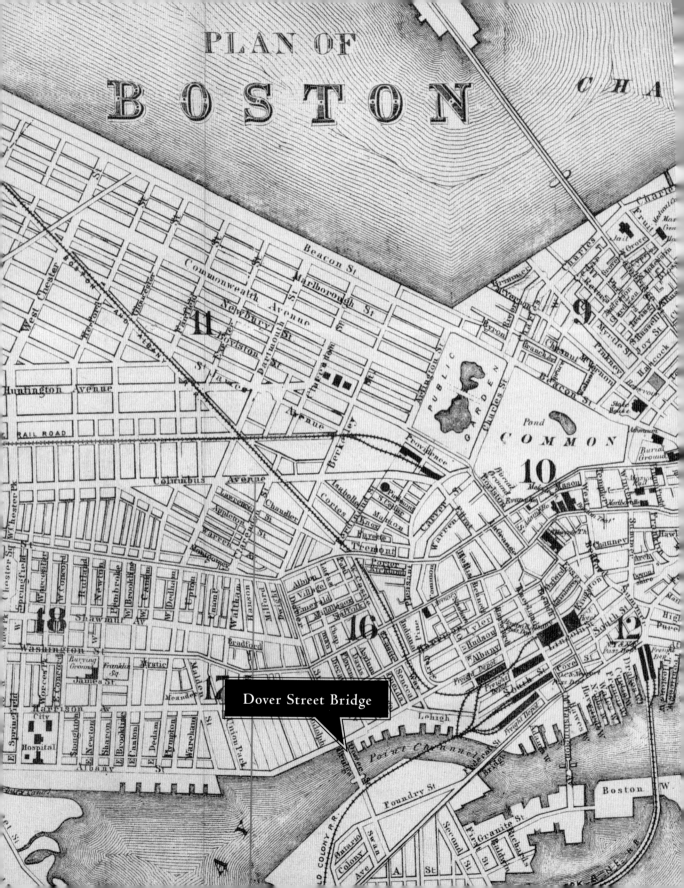

PLAN OF BOSTON

Dover Street Bridge

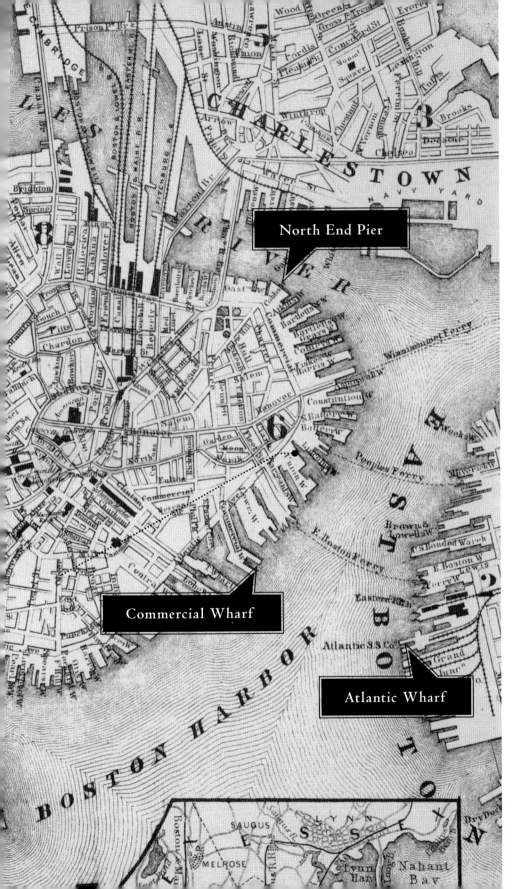

Dover Street Bridge: Reverend Rufus Tobey's inspiration for the Boston Floating Hospital came from watching desperate parents bring their ailing children to the bridge for fresh, clean air.

Commercial Wharf: Families lined up at Commercial Wharf from 1894 to 1906, waiting to be admitted to board the *Clifford*. The Floating's first dock was situated near the North End, where so many of the families who needed the Floating lived.

Atlantic Wharf: The *Clifford* spent its winters at Atlantic Wharf, undergoing routine maintenance and awaiting its summers on the harbor.

North End Pier: In 1906 the North End Pier became the Floating's home, until a fire destroyed the ship in 1927.

PROLOGUE

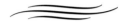

The second half of the nineteenth century was a time of change and upheaval worldwide. In America—with the aftermath of the Civil War—it was a time of both great prosperity and great poverty. An era of social and scientific revolution was about to occur with unprecedented advances in technology and productivity. A shrinking geopolitical stage brought countries together—sometimes peacefully and occasionally under the threat of war. Innovation and collaboration would eventually draw scientists and physicians together to invent anesthesia, identify infectious agents, and reduce maternal mortality. Despite these advances, at the end of the century, life continued to remain a challenge. Infant mortality was still high, infectious diseases and epidemics were common, and medicine was largely unchanged by advances in other fields.

In the 1890s, Boston was a microcosm of this world. An economic depression known as the "Panic of 1893," triggered by a fall in gold reserves, disrupted confidence in the value of U.S. currency. Five hundred banks and sixteen thousand businesses failed, resulting in a depression that lasted until 1897.[1] Unemployment in Massachusetts went from 1.51 percent in 1892 to 8.51 percent in 1893. In Boston, ten thousand people received work relief assistance from various citizen committees between 1893 and 1894.[2] The poor immigrants arriving from Europe felt the effects of this depression disproportionately.

The root causes of the enormous influx of immigrants from Europe and Asia to the coasts of the United States (Boston and New York on the East and San Francisco on the West) were large-scale economic failures, famine, political unrest, and targeted persecution of specific ethnic groups.

In striking contrast, artistic creativity exploded in the 1890s. Nellie Melba sang in Gounod's *Romeo and Juliet* at the Boston Opera House in March 1894. *The Jungle Book* was published, and, that same year, a twenty-year-old Robert Frost sold his first poem, "My Butterfly." George Bernard Shaw's *Arms and the Man* was a huge success. In Spain, Pablo Picasso was already painting at the age of twelve.

In 1894, New England Telephone and Telegraph installed the first battery-operated telephone switchboard in Lexington, Massachusetts. William Kennedy Dickson received a patent for motion picture film, and Karl Benz of Germany received the U.S. patent for a gasoline-driven automobile. In 1897, Boston opened the first subway system in the country, and people soon grew used to riding in a trolley car that moved through a tunnel.

Layered upon this was the emerging realization that the health of a nation was, to a great extent, dependent on the health of its children. But for poor children in Boston, health was frequently an elusive goal.

Against this backdrop of change and progress, The Boston Floating Hospital, affectionately called "the Floating," embarked on its 1894 maiden voyage. The following pages will take you into this exciting time, into an era that was filled with the promise of the next century while still burdened with the problems of the past. The Floating can be seen as a symbol of that time as it contributed to the development of medicine and pioneered many of the new approaches to social welfare and the delivery of health care services that were to become hallmarks of the twentieth century.

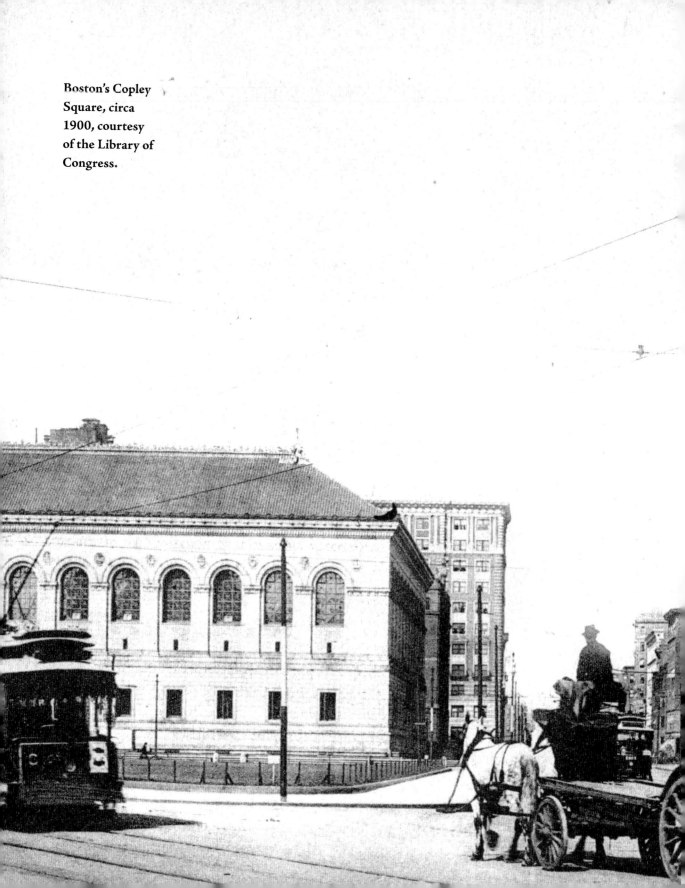

Boston's Copley
Square, circa
1900, courtesy
of the Library of
Congress.

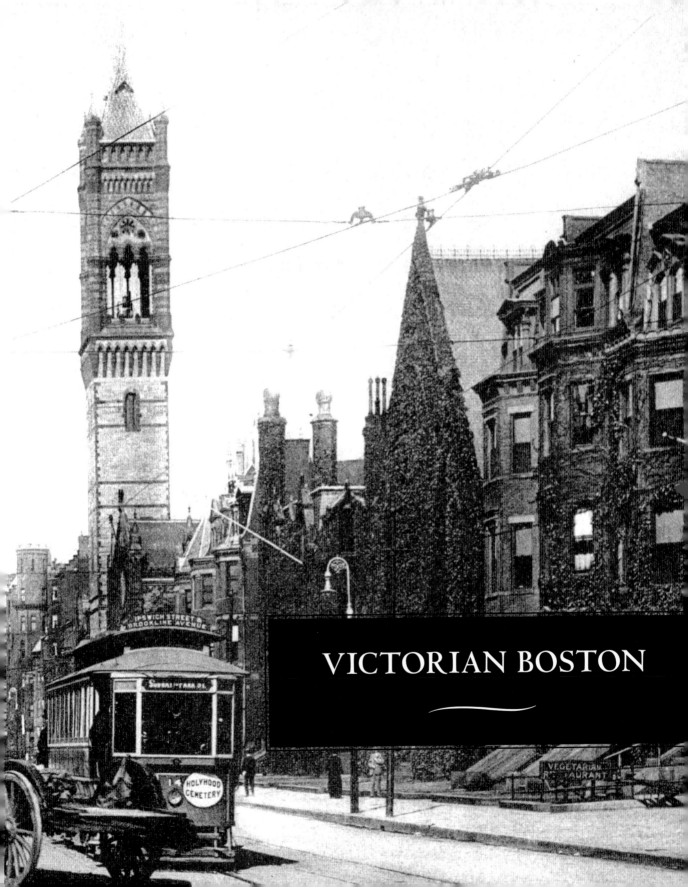

VICTORIAN BOSTON

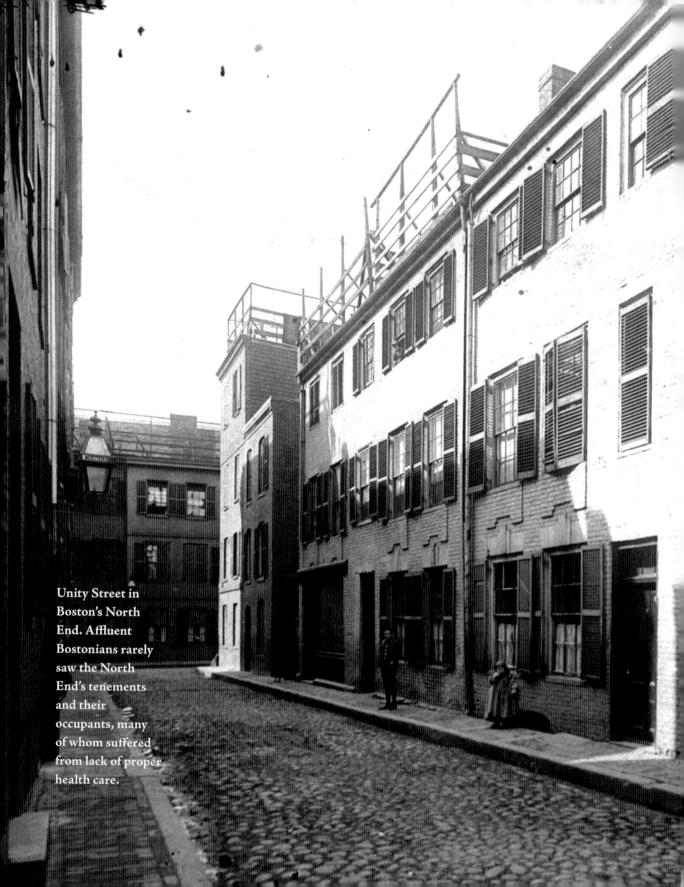

Unity Street in
Boston's North
End. Affluent
Bostonians rarely
saw the North
End's tenements
and their
occupants, many
of whom suffered
from lack of proper
health care.

VICTORIAN BOSTON

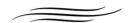

In 1842, Charles Dickens traveled to Boston and visited the Perkins Institute for the Blind and several other institutions serving poor, handicapped children. The creator of Tiny Tim and David Copperfield was impressed with the charitable impulses that had led Boston's citizens to care for these unfortunate youngsters. And he found Boston itself pleasing: "The city is a beautiful one and cannot fail, I should imagine, to impress all strangers very favorably. The private dwelling houses are, for the most part, large and elegant; the shops extremely good and the public buildings handsome. The State House is built upon the summit of a hill, which rises gradually at first and afterwards by a steep ascent almost from the water's edge. In front is a green enclosure, called the Common. The site is beautiful and from the top there is a charming panoramic view of the whole town and neighborhood." [1]

Boston's most generous hostesses entertained the famous British guest, and he roamed about the city's graceful streets. But from the heights of Beacon Hill, Dickens did not get a panoramic view of the "whole town and neighborhood." Hidden behind the houses of the Boston Brahmins were the slums where the city's poor working people lived. Thousands subsisted in crowded, unsanitary tenements, which were freezing cold in winter and unbearably hot in summer. Hunger, poverty, and disease were the companions of those who lived there. Boston may have been a modern-day Athens for the well-educated people who lived on Beacon Hill, but for the poor of the city, Calcutta would have been a more apt comparison.

The Irish potato famine of the 1840s resulted in a flood of immigration that swelled the population of Boston and established its large, flourishing Irish community. The Irish weren't alone; Italians, Poles, and Germans also poured into Boston. By mid-century, Americans from impoverished rural communities flocked to the city to work in the newly established leather factories and in the mills in Lowell and Lawrence. The seaport gave employment to able-bodied seamen; the fishing industry flourished. In fact, Gallops Island welcomed so many immigrants from 1860 to 1880 that the Statue of Liberty came very close to being placed in Boston Harbor!

Some lucky young women found jobs as maids and cooks in the mansions on Beacon Hill. While they were able to escape the intolerable conditions of the poor neighborhoods, these women still lived in tiny rooms, were paid little, and worked long hours ironing, cooking, and cleaning for the large families that inhabited the posh sections of town. Aside from these live-in maids, most of the new immigrants lived in sub-standard housing far from the eyes of Boston's wealthy.

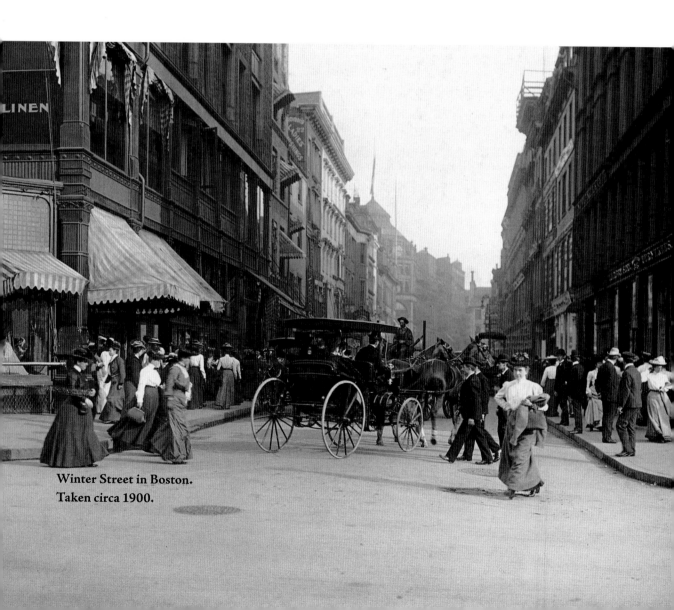

Winter Street in Boston.
Taken circa 1900.

INFANT MORTALITY

In 1850, the U.S. population was twenty-three million with 42 percent of the population under fifteen years of age; by 1900 it had grown to seventy-six million with 34 percent under fifteen years of age. In 1890 the city of Boston had a population of nearly four hundred and fifty thousand. Like other urban areas, its population grew rapidly, and by the end of the century there were five hundred and sixty thousand inhabitants.[2]

From 1855 to 1865, 96.2 children out of every 1,000 in Boston died before they were five years old.[3] Lemuel Shattuck (1793–1859), a Massachusetts public health pioneer and innovator, wrote in 1845 about one poor section of Boston that "children seem literally "born to die."[4] The rise in deaths was due to diseases that found a breeding ground in the poorly ventilated, unsanitary surroundings of the urban slums that had sprung up to house the thousands of new immigrants. These included diphtheria, measles, scarlet fever, whooping cough, cholera infantum, dysentery, and a host of other maladies ravaging the poorest children of the city.

ATTITUDES TOWARD THE POOR

In most areas of the United States, private doctors treated the well-to-do in the patients' own homes; only the poor went to hospitals when they were sick.[5] Indeed, hospitals were considered unsafe, as "hospitalism," the incidence of hospital-originated fevers and infections, was a genuine threat until these institutions began to practice methods of antisepsis.[6] During the Civil War, hospital care was provided for wounded soldiers for the first time on a mass scale, but once the war was over, those who could afford it continued to see their private doctors in their offices or at home. Even Florence Nightingale declared that cleanliness and good food at home were better than hospital care.

The poor were cared for in charity hospitals that had developed from almshouses. In these institutions, the conventional wisdom was that there was something about being poor that caused the indigent to fall ill, and this prejudice was reflected in the way charity patients were treated.[7]

The boards of directors of these hospitals, not doctors, decreed who could be admitted, and although their members thought they operated from a sense of noblesse oblige, they preferred to provide care only to the "worthy" poor. For example, the managers of the Boston Children's Hospital (founded in 1869) acknowledged in their third annual report that their patients came from "the very lowest; from abodes of drunkenness and vice in almost every form, where the most depressing and corrupting influences were acting both on the body and the mind."[8] Poor children were considered good prospects for changing the dreadful lifestyles of their elders. The board of directors of the Boston Children's Hospital saw it as its duty to help "the child soul to lift itself out of the mud in which it had been born to assert its native purity in spite of unfortunate surroundings."[9]

To this end, visiting hours in many hospitals were so restricted that the parents of young patients were virtually unable to see their children. This isolation gave the upstanding men and women of the hospital's "visiting committees" the opportunity to teach the children better living habits, cleanliness, and especially lessons about morals in the hope that they would transmit these lessons to their parents when they were released back to their care.

CHILDREN'S MEDICINE

Until the 1870s, hospitals in America did not recognize the various specialties of medicine. In 1908, there were not more than thirty doctors in the country who exclusively specialized in the care of children.

The Massachusetts General Hospital had established a dermatology clinic in 1869, and by 1873, dermatology, nervous diseases, diseases of the throat, and ophthalmology had become separate departments at that hospital. Children's diseases did not have their own branch of medicine until the last decades of the nineteenth century. Even then, most children were seen by the doctors who treated their mothers. Pediatrics was nothing more than an "appendage of obstetrics."

Until the nineteenth century, children were treated as if they were just smaller versions of adults, potential grown-ups who needed molding and discipline. By the turn of the twentieth century, these attitudes were slowly changing. In 1898, the *Archives of Pediatrics* noted:

"To the student of sociology, one of the most notable features of the past few decades is the growing attention bestowed upon children. The thought now devoted to them would amaze our ancestors of three generations ago. Child-study has become one of great importance. Thousands of men and women are being trained in scores of normal schools for the one purpose of instructing the young, for the work of a teacher is now believed to be one demanding extensive and peculiar education. Volumes are written annually for children and of children, while journals and magazines of the same character have increased a hundred-fold. The children are apparently considered a far more important factor in every household than they were fifty years ago. It is at least a fact that they receive more attention and are brought into much greater prominence. The average child of to-day has a score of toys where his grandfather had one."[10]

Still, most doctors did not recognize the special medical needs of children even though they were aware that the mortality rate among children was much higher than that of adults. That a certain number of children died before their first birthdays was simply a fact of life, and accurate infant mortality figures were not available until accurate birth records began to be kept.

In Boston between 1840 and 1845, 40 percent of all deaths were among children under the age of five.[11] In fact, deaths among children between the ages of five and nineteen were higher in the mid-nineteenth century than at the end of the eighteenth century. This rise in child mortality was due to the growth of cities where crowded conditions, poor hygiene, and contaminated food provided a perfect environment for the spread of those diseases to which children were particularly vulnerable.

In 1841, Shattuck commented on the "increasing and alarming mortality" among infants. He attributed this to "more luxury and effeminacy in both sexes which may have produced children with constitutional debility and feeble health." More accurately, he also acknowledged "nursing and feeding of children with improper food is another cause. The influence of bad air in confined, badly located and filthy houses is another and perhaps the greatest."[12]

The mortality of foundlings under the age of one year in some almshouses was as high as 97 percent in the middle of the nineteenth century, and this "alarming mortality" led to a demand for hospitals for poor children.[13] The first pediatric hospital was founded in Philadelphia in 1855, and the Boston Children's Hospital was established in 1869. Like other hospitals, these early children's hospitals served only the poor. By 1889, when Babies Hospital was founded in New York, there were fewer than half a dozen general hospitals with wards for infants.[14] By the turn of the century, more than two dozen children's hospitals had been established and 64 of the country's 119 medical schools had a special chair for pediatrics.

Children's diseases were not even mentioned in the Harvard Medical School announcement until 1871, when Francis Minot was appointed assistant professor of the theory and practice of medicine and clinical lecturer in the diseases of women and children. In 1888, Thomas Morgan Rotch (1849-1914) was appointed assistant professor of the diseases of children at Harvard Medical School; in 1893 he was promoted to professor of the diseases of children, and in 1903 his title was changed to "Professor of Pediatrics." His was the first real professorship of pediatrics in the country.[15]

The physician who worked most effectively to establish pediatrics as an important branch of American medicine was Abraham Jacobi, a German refugee who organized the first children's clinic in New York City at the New York Medical College (not connected to the modern medical school of the same name) in 1860. He worked at every hospital in New York but concentrated on the Jews Hospital (later known as Mount Sinai), where he set up the first outpatient pediatric clinic in 1874. In 1878, Mount Sinai Hospital established the first department of pediatrics in an American general hospital. In 1880, Jacobi was the organizer and became the chairman of the first section on pediatrics of the American Medical Association; Rotch was its first secretary. [16]

Jacobi, always ahead of his time, was opposed to the constant use of calomel (a "purgative" that induced vomiting and a favorite among doctors treating infants) and was once reprimanded from the pulpit for advocating that children should be undressed in hot weather.

Despite the academic attention pediatrics received, it was of little interest to general practitioners for many years. Perhaps this was because there was very little doctors could do in those days to treat or cure childhood diseases. Diphtheria anti-toxin was introduced in Boston in 1894, but it was not widely distributed, and the other childhood illnesses could not be prevented. Measles, scarlet fever, whooping cough, and mumps were rampant and deadly diseases in those days; physicians were nearly helpless in treating them and most of the other ailments plaguing children.

The impact of science on the practice of medicine was negligible as the nineteenth century ended. There were very few laboratories to investigate the causes for pediatric diseases, to search for cures, or to study tissue samples or cultures from sick children. The medical tools and resources of the time consisted of primitive or dangerous medications whose side effects were not well understood. For these reasons, the therapies most often recommended involved fresh air and sunshine, and these natural remedies remained commonly used weapons in the treatment of disease until well into the twentieth century.

While American medicine was slow to accept the germ theory, by the 1880s it was generally accepted that bacteria in milk were responsible for intestinal diseases of children. Most doctors advocated for the wider availability of pure milk for infants. Unable to do much for their patients, doctors concentrated on adjusting what infants were fed and finding foods they could digest. Indeed, pediatricians were popularly referred to as "baby feeders."

It was debilitating poverty, prejudices against the poor, and insufficient knowledge of children's medicine that provided the backdrop for the inception and execution of an idea that would change how poor children were treated by physicians, ultimately revolutionizing how the medical community viewed pediatrics overall.

The origins of the Floating were simple and modest. Its founders wanted a practical solution to a pervasive problem: poor children were dying by the hundreds during the summer from intestinal diseases that were rampant in the crowded slums. The doctors of that time were only beginning to forge weapons against these intestinal illnesses, but they knew that if children could get into the fresh air, away from their environment, if they could be given good food and compassionate medical care, they would have a better chance to recover. Of these three prescriptions, the most readily available was fresh air, but for a variety of reasons it was often difficult for poor parents to take advantage of this simple directive.

It was not a doctor but a Congregational minister who had the imagination and vision to understand that a healthy atmosphere and medical care could be combined on a hospital boat that could venture out onto the water and expose its passengers to cool breezes and sea air. On board, as far from the city and its squalor as possible, a staff of doctors and nurses would see to their patients' medical needs. Luckily, in addition to his vision, this man possessed the determination that made his dream come true. In just a few years, a small barge developed into a pediatric hospital ship internationally known for its success in treating childhood diseases and its research facilities. In time, it far surpassed the modest aspirations of its founders as it developed into an important land-based pediatric teaching hospital as well.

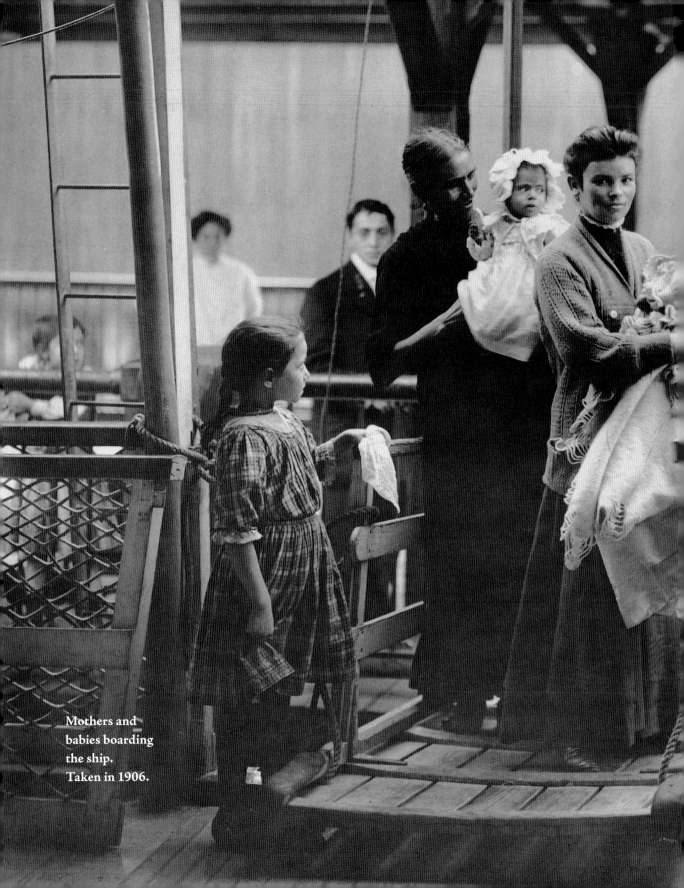

Mothers and
babies boarding
the ship.
Taken in 1906.

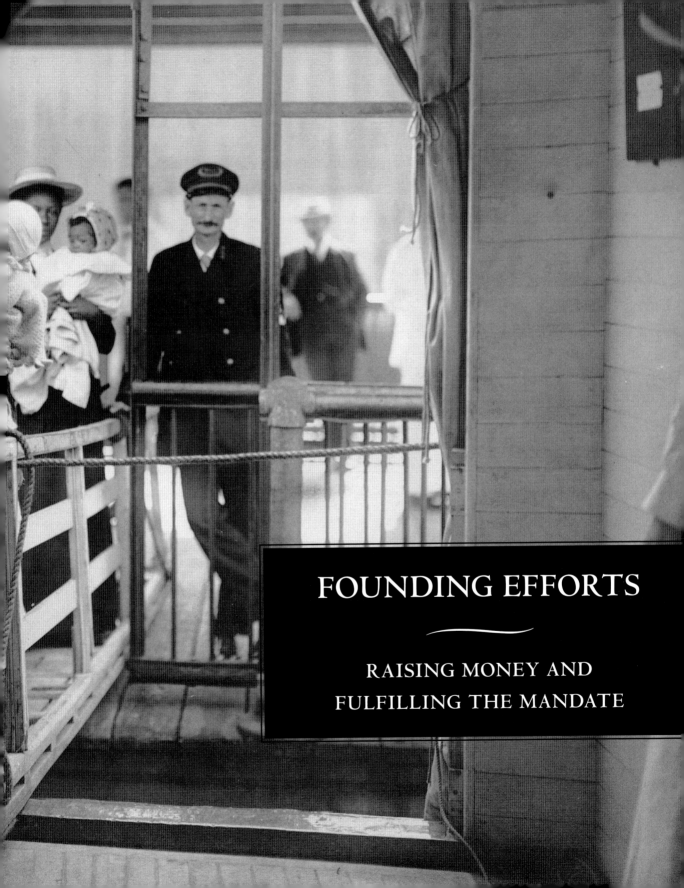

FOUNDING EFFORTS

RAISING MONEY AND
FULFILLING THE MANDATE

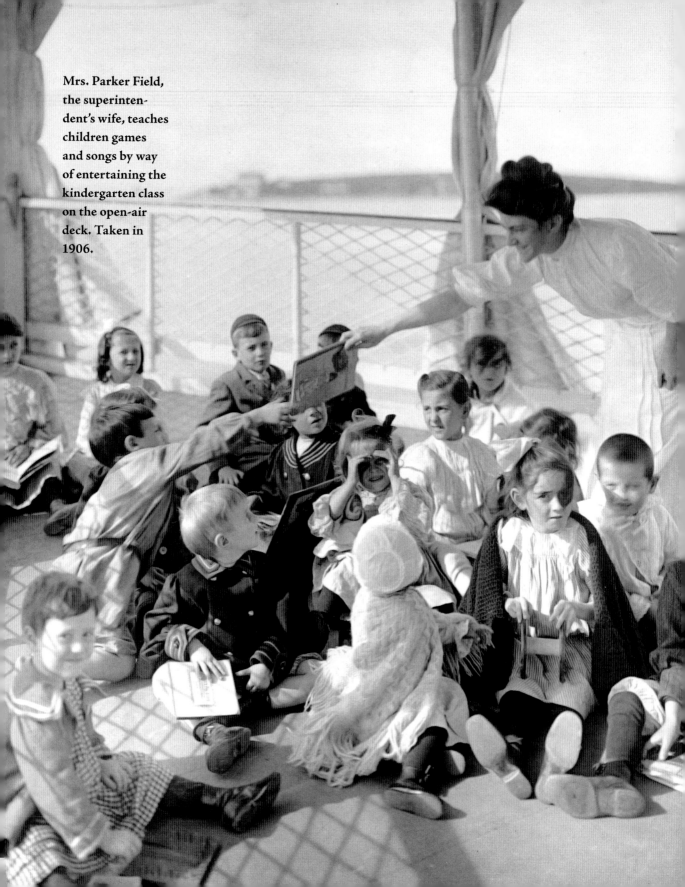

Mrs. Parker Field, the superintendent's wife, teaches children games and songs by way of entertaining the kindergarten class on the open-air deck. Taken in 1906.

FOUNDING EFFORTS
RAISING MONEY AND FULFILLING THE MANDATE

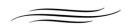

On the morning of July 25, 1894,[1] those citizens of Boston who regularly took an early morning stroll near Snow's Wharf were astonished to see the barge *Clifford* being towed out into the harbor. Typically, the *Clifford* returned to her berth at midnight, after a night during which her decks were crowded with revelers out for a romantic cruise. But now, where deck chairs and dining tables had stood, there were hammocks and cots. The bar and the bandstand had been replaced by hospital gear. If they had been able to go below decks, those who saw the *Clifford* that morning would have noted the lower decks had been divided into wards and a dispensary. From the roof of the *Clifford's* cabin hung a twenty-foot-long white banner emblazoned with green crosses.

The barge no longer resembled a pleasure craft. Between midnight and its 9:00 a.m. departure time, the *Clifford* had been transformed into The Boston Floating Hospital.

The passengers had begun to assemble at 8:00 a.m. It must have been a noisy, chaotic scene. Women, holding the hands of restless toddlers and carrying infants in their arms, stood in a haphazard formation that stretched along the pier. Eventually, they were welcomed on board by a doctor who took the red slips of paper that served as their tickets from their hands. These slips had been issued to the Associated Charities, a welfare agency serving the poor, the dispensaries, the hospitals, and many of the city's doctors. When signed by a physician, the slips certified that the baby was sick (but not with a contagious disease like whooping cough or diphtheria). When the gangplank was taken up, in addition to the mothers and their children, the passengers included a staff of volunteers: two physicians, several medical students, and two nurses assisted by a group of women. With Captain E.W. Sears at the helm of the barge, and the tug, *Leader*, pulling it along, the Floating began her maiden voyage.

FOUNDING FATHERS

Who was behind the *Clifford*'s transformation? Two men, in particular, saw the growing needs of the poor and their children. Reverend Rufus Babcock Tobey and his assistant, Lewis Freeman, were the driving force behind the Floating. Supported by Boston's charitable organizations, Reverend Tobey and Mr. Freeman, along with Edward Everett Hale, began a crusade for those who needed medical services but could not afford them.

Tobey

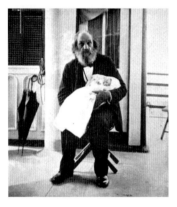

Reverend Tobey[2] was the assistant pastor of the Berkeley Temple, situated at Berkeley Street and Warren Avenue close to the city's poorest neighborhoods. It was a so-called Institutional Church, where charity was a sacred duty and devotion to God was expressed in good works. Like the Settlement Houses in New York City, the Berkeley Temple functioned as a community center, a social service agency to which people with few other options could appeal for help with the problems they faced in their lives. The origin of the Floating could be traced to the Reverend Tobey's profound dedication to aiding the poor of the city of Boston.

In the summer months, busy late into the night at the Berkeley Temple, Reverend Tobey and his assistant, Mr. Freeman, would walk across the Dover Street Bridge (or South Bridge) to the station where Reverend Tobey caught

Reverend Rufus Tobey with a small patient in his arms. Taken in 1899.

———

The Dover Street Bridge opened in 1805 and was a fashionable promenade offering an attractive view of the town. By the time Reverend Tobey walked across the bridge in the 1890s, it had lost its appeal because of the building of the railroad and the development of the South Cove area. *Amerique septentrionale etat de Massachusetts: Boston from the South Boston Bridge. Adam, Victor, 1801-1866, lithographer. Paris. [Printed and] published by Henry Gaugain, 1828.*

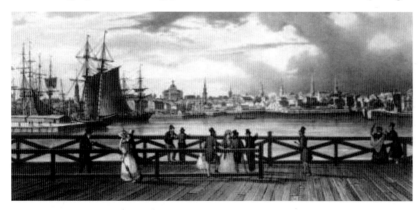

the train to his home in Quincy. On those hot nights, Reverend Tobey and Mr. Freeman encountered poor fathers and mothers, often with sick children in their arms, trying to find a breath of fresh air. The children of the poor were dying every summer of acute intestinal infections called "cholera infantum." The medical profession was unable to do much for babies suffering from this terrible disease. The only prescription at the time was good food, and in particular, pure milk, but these commodities were not readily available to the poor.

But doctors also believed that fresh air could have a beneficial effect on the health of these children. And since fresh air was available to everyone, parents were taking their sick children as close to the harbor as they could. The air at the harbor was a bit cooler than in the stifling slums, but a walk on this bridge over the steaming railroad yards was certainly not what the doctors had in mind. Reverend Tobey was so moved by these people trying desperately to help their children that he decided then and there to open a hospital on the water. Reverend Tobey's vision of a hospital that would float in Boston Harbor for the benefit of the poor soon became legend.

In fact, the plight of poor families had long engaged Reverend Tobey as he worked at the Berkeley Temple, and for some time, he had been involved with several organizations that were trying to provide respite from the summer heat for poor families. No doubt the sight of those poor parents and their sick children moved Reverend Tobey deeply, and seeing them on every hot summer night must have strengthened the resolve that something needed to be done. Indeed, Reverend Tobey had been actively working with the Unitarian minister, author, and famous orator, Edward Everett Hale for some time to find a solution to this problem.

Known today primarily for his short story "The Man Without A Country," Hale was then equally famous for his novel *Ten Times One is Ten*, a parable demonstrating his thesis that if one person could inspire ten others to do good works, those ten would each involve another ten, and those ten would recruit ten others, until a large network was formed. He wrote that if ten workers for good were multiplied by ten every three years, at the end of twenty-seven years, the whole world would accept faith, hope, and love as the rule of life.

A letter from the Ten Times One Society. Written May 15, 1897.

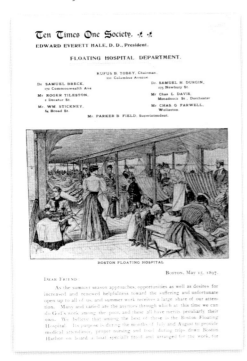

In response to the book's message, Ten Times One Societies and Lend A Hand Clubs had been formed all over New England. These charitable organizations had as their motto the admonition: "Look up and not down, look forward and not back, look out and not in. Lend a Hand."

Reverend Tobey and Hale had worked together in the Seashore Homes Association, a group dedicated to providing short summer vacations for the city's poorest mothers and children. The association was also discussing plans for a hospital at the shore where the curative properties of salt air could be readily available to the sick. But while Seashore Homes was able to board families for brief vacations in the country, Reverend Tobey and Hale had become discouraged about the prospects of raising the funds necessary to establish the Seashore Hospital.

It was around that time that Reverend Tobey heard about the hull of a steamboat that had been converted into a hospital ship in New York City. Under the auspices of the St. John's Guild, The Floating Hospital of New York, *The Emma Abbott,* had been making three trips a week since 1875 during "the heated term," taking mothers and children out into New York Harbor for the day. Doctors on board treated the sick children or sent them to hospitals after the day's trip was over, and everyone benefited from an outing in the sea air on what was essentially an outpatient clinic on the water. Reverend Tobey was struck with the vision of a similar boat taking Boston's sick children out into the harbor, and he set out to translate this dream into reality.

During the winter of 1893, Reverend Tobey, Hale, and Dr. Francis H. Brown (one of the founders of the Boston Children's Hospital) tried to sell the idea of a floating hospital to various groups in Boston without success. Reverend Tobey even arranged for John P. Faure, chairman of the St. John's Guild, to give an illustrated lecture about the New York boat to groups associated with Boston's charities. Although a prominent charity called "The Monday Evening Club" endorsed the plan, no one was eager to take on the responsibility of launching such a venture. Reverend Tobey was told that he was the best man for the job because of his experience at the Berkeley Temple, but his work there was already keeping him fully occupied. His office was crowded from early morning until late at night with needy people seeking his help.

At this time Reverend Tobey learned that the *Clifford,* a barge owned by Boston Shoe dealer Edward Wildes, was available for charter. Built in Bangor, Maine, in 1876, the barge weighed 237.7 tons and was 131.9 feet long and 26.5 feet wide. It had two decks and a cabin. Reverend Tobey thought that this was just the kind of vessel he needed. With the help of The Monday Evening Club and using the funds he had on hand, Reverend Tobey chartered the barge. He planned to use the first trip to demonstrate the need, as well as the feasibility, of floating a hospital on the waters of Boston Harbor.

Freeman

That Mr. Freeman and Reverend Tobey should have come together is amazing since they were from altogether different backgrounds. In addition to being from different social strata, Mr. Freeman was of African-American descent—though this was not how he identified himself. As his wife, who was white, put it, Mr. Freeman wanted "to be taken as a man who through his own efforts has achieved what he has achieved. Let him be valued only as an American in the true sense of the word." Despite their different circumstances, it was Mr. Freeman who found Reverend Tobey, and the two men forged a partnership that was not only unique for the time but also inspiring.

Mr. Freeman,[3] born in Washington D.C., was the son of an attaché to a Central American diplomatic delegation and an African-American mother who was a singer with musical ambitions for her son. Mr. Freeman was five years old and visiting his grandmother in Alexandria, Virginia, when the state voted to secede from the Union. He and his grandmother were among the last people to escape from the city ahead of the federal troops.

After the Civil War, when Mr. Freeman was thirteen and living in Washington D.C., a teacher named Bartlett took an interest in him. He persuaded Mr. Freeman's mother to let him take the boy on a summer trip up north so that he could teach him shorthand. They traveled to Baltimore, Philadelphia, and Boston, where he proclaimed, "That's the city where I want to live." In Maine, their next stop, Mr. Bartlett began the shorthand lessons.

The Clifford being pulled by its tugboat. As a barge, the Clifford was unable to move through the harbor on its own. This tugboat navigated the waters while doctors and nurses tended to the patients until the Clifford anchored for the night. Taken in 1899.

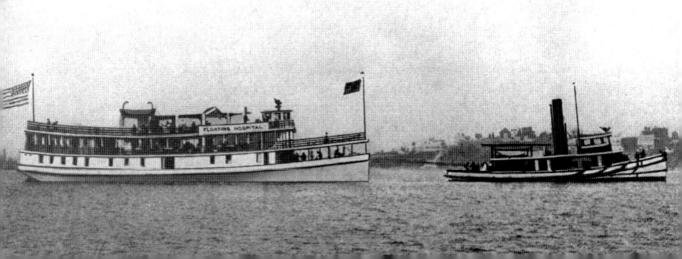

For Mr. Freeman, shorthand proved to be a valuable skill. He augmented his fifteen-dollar-a-month income as a messenger for several senators by doing stenographic work in his spare time.

Later, Mr. Freeman became a secretary to a Washington lawyer and then worked for the Honorable William A. Russell of Lawrence, Massachusetts, for three years. He resigned because of an illness, but when he recovered in 1890, he finally made his way to his favorite city: Boston. Soon after he arrived, he walked into the Berkeley Temple and was hired as Reverend Tobey's clerk and assistant.

While the contemporary accounts of the Floating hardly mention Mr. Freeman, his service to the Floating spanned the entire history of the hospital on the boat. Indeed, there is reason to believe that Mr. Freeman wrote or edited many of the early annual reports. G. Loring Briggs, the hospital's business manager from 1906 to 1927, often remarked on "the faithfulness and ability of Mr. Freeman."

Mr. Freeman had the complete confidence of Reverend Tobey, who put him in charge of the boat's finances and the everyday operation of the vessel from the start. No person was more devoted to the Floating than Mr. Freeman. As he told Elsie Briggs, "I look on my whole life, almost from birth, as a preparation for my service to The Boston Floating Hospital."

A drawing of the early days on the Clifford. This image was used in newspapers and fundraising materials.

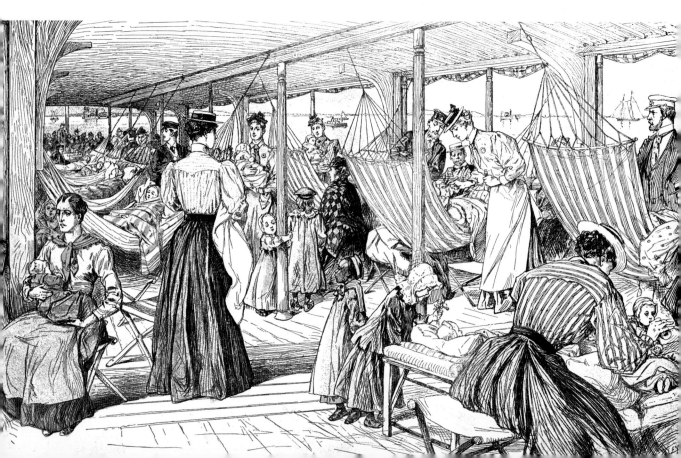

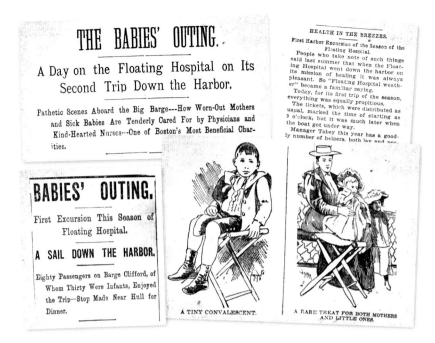

THE BABIES' OUTING.

A Day on the Floating Hospital on Its Second Trip Down the Harbor.

Pathetic Scenes Aboard the Big Barge---How Worn-Out Mothers and Sick Babies Are Tenderly Cared For by Physicians and Kind-Hearted Nurses---One of Boston's Most Beneficial Charities.

BABIES' OUTING.

First Excursion This Season of Floating Hospital.

A SAIL DOWN THE HARBOR.

Eighty Passengers on Barge Clifford, of Whom Thirty Were Infants, Enjoyed the Trip—Stop Made Near Hull for Dinner.

A TINY CONVALESCENT.

A RARE TREAT FOR BOTH MOTHERS AND LITTLE ONES.

HEALTH IN THE BREEZES.

First Harbor Excursion of the Season of the Floating Hospital.

People who take note of such things said last summer that when the Floating Hospital went down the harbor on its mission of healing it was always pleasant. So "Floating Hospital weather" became a familiar saying. Today, for its first trip of the season, everything was equally propitious.

The tickets, which were distributed as usual, marked the time of starting as 9 o'clock, but it was much later when the boat got under way.

Manager Tobey this year has a good-ly number of helpers, both lay and pro-

EARLY FUNDRAISING EFFORTS

While most of Reverend Tobey's visitors to the Berkeley Temple were looking for help, he had other visitors as well. Mrs. Florence Hunt, a reporter for the *Boston Herald*, stopped in regularly in search of good human-interest stories. When Reverend Tobey happened to mention his idea of a floating hospital, she sensed a great story—just the sort of thing to which her readers would respond. Her article in the morning paper [4] gave the impression that Reverend Tobey, on the verge of launching a floating hospital, was looking for funds. In the days following the publication of the story, a small flood of contributions for the as-yet non-existent Boston Floating Hospital arrived in Reverend Tobey's office. The embarrassed reverend returned most of the gifts but was left with about four hundred dollars of anonymous contributions.

The Floating's maiden voyage, which had been planned only as a demonstration of need and feasibility, was described by the press in glowing terms complete with touching (and somewhat sentimental, perhaps even slightly condescending) anecdotes about poor, sick babies and a description of the barge itself. Stories about the Floating often contained paragraphs like this one:

"There was enough (fresh air) to go around twice for every pale, peaked little sufferer there, and then enough left over for the tired, hollow eyed mothers and the rollicking imps who came along because they could not be left at home ... no one who saw those children go on the boat in the morning and come off again in the afternoon, can doubt that they went away with a spot of sunshine in their little lives, brighter than any they are likely to get hereafter." [5]

While today's tastes would consider the prose too flowery and many would object to the patronizing tone, these stories inspired sympathy for the impoverished families and support for the hospital.

After word of The Boston Floating Hospital's first trip came out in the papers, enough money was donated for the *Clifford* to make four more trips that first year. Having proved that health agencies and doctors would send patients to the Floating and that the boat was a good environment for treating them, Reverend Tobey set the goal for the following year at twenty trips.

The cost of each trip the first year was $246.35. Donations totaled $1,962.68, and at the end of the summer there was a $700 surplus in the treasury. By the fall of 1894, looking back on what they had accomplished during their first season, Reverend Tobey and the doctors expanded their mandate. They wanted to raise enough money for the summer of 1895 to offer "intelligent instructions for the mothers, with proper food and medicine and constant care for three or four hundred poor, sick and helpless babies" on each trip.

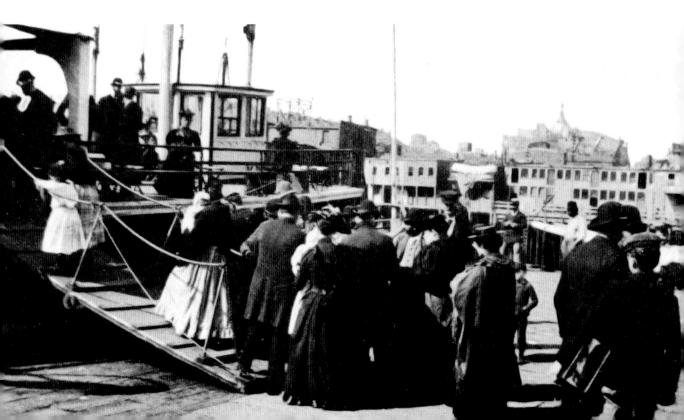

Embarking on the
Clifford *in 1895*

The Seashore Homes project that had engaged Reverend Tobey and Hale had been in existence for more than two decades when the Floating was launched. In its first year, Seashore Homes cared for 140 children; the Floating, however, served 1,100 children and 650 mothers during its first season in 1894. In a historical sketch published in the 1898 annual report, Hale reported that they "watched the successes of this enterprise with profound interest," adding that Seashore Homes eventually "dissolved their own corporation as unnecessary in view of the larger opportunities afforded by the daily trips of our barge." [6]

In 1895, Reverend Tobey severed his connection to the Berkeley Temple and opened an office at 198 Dartmouth Street, where he devoted his full time to the Floating.[7] Mr. Freeman continued as his assistant and became the Floating's manager, handling the office work and overseeing the finances as bookkeeper. The hospital was now organized as The Boston Floating Hospital Corporation with Reverend Tobey as its first chairman.

The second season of the Floating built on the success of the first. Opening day on July 12, 1895, was timed to coincide with the annual convention of the Christian Endeavor Society, a charitable organization that was one of the Floating's chief supporters. The members joined mothers and patients on the first

CLARK

In 1896 a new fundraising idea was introduced. For a gift of $100, generous patrons could name a day's trip in honor of anyone they chose. The first such contribution came from Mr. Benjamin Cutler Clark, president of Pearson Cordage Company, manufacturers of cordage and binder twine, located in Roxbury. He had previously served as ambassador to Haiti and was a well-known philanthropist. Mr. Clark named the first trip for Edward Everett Hale.[1]

Mr. Clark was described in the Boston Advertiser as possessing "a magnetic personality, a whole souled cordial manner and a frank sincerity in his smiling face which at once won him the confidence of every man, woman, and child. He is tall and broad shouldered with a fine physique. His face is always smooth. He is always well and carefully dressed with a boutonniere of fresh flowers. A day with the Floating Hospital children seems equally enjoyed by them and him. His pockets are full of sweets and his arms full of flowers. When he has given them out he gets a new supply and two hours after starting the boat looks like a full blown flower garden."[2]

The Herald for Sunday, July 11, 1896 also described the scene as Mr. Clark arrived on board for the trip he had again named for Edward Everett Hale: "Mr. Benjamin C. Clark, the Haytian (sic) Consul said 'I trust there will be flowers, children and poetry in heaven. For I think heaven would surely be more beautiful with all these additions' as he moved about in his cheerful way and distributing roses, sweet peas and carnations among the sick little ones swinging in their hammocks." For many years it was a Floating tradition that the generous Mr. Clark would endow the first day's sailing.

trip, a gesture calculated to encourage contributions and to show the membership how the hospital worked.

By its second year, the Floating had acquired a surgical ward and could report a number of successful operations. But even in 1901—by which time there was a fully equipped operating room on board—the directors did not consider surgery to be one of the major objectives of the hospital because "many other institutions were available for such cases." The primary role for the Floating was to care for poor children who could not be treated for their summer diseases anywhere else. For example, Boston's Infants' Hospital [8] closed during the summer months because it was unable to cope with these illnesses. It simply could not handle the volume of patients and did not have the supplies and clean milk necessary to treat these ailments.

While the Floating soon became a well-known institution and a favorite charity of many of Boston's citizens, in 1895 a group of unscrupulous men approached its board of directors with a fundraising suggestion. They proposed to mount a benefit musical performance of *Cinderella*. The money would come from the sale of program ads to local businesses with all the proceeds to go to the Floating. It sounded like a wonderful plan, but it turned out to be a scam. The performance took place, but as the newspaper accounts put it, the "shrewd speculators" pocketed the funds and left the hospital three hundred dollars in the red. The sale of the extravagant costumes that had added so much to the production settled the bill.[9]

The papers gave this "scandal" a great deal of space because the Floating was not the only institution that had been so cheated. While the *Cinderella* affair did not permanently harm the reputation or the future of the Floating (because Reverend Tobey himself was not implicated in the scandal), the directors vowed to ban any future collection of funds by unknown organizations. In this way, they would be able

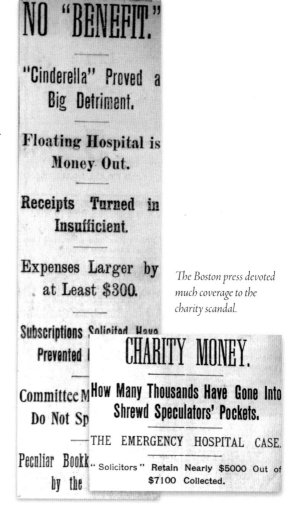

The Boston press devoted much coverage to the charity scandal.

to guarantee that every cent contributed to the Floating would be used for the patients. The hospital directors often repeated this rule, warning that "no collector of funds is authorized under any consideration."

From the outset, it was part of the Floating's philosophy to be supported by contributions from the public. Even before the boat was launched, the hospital was a pet project of Boston's newspapers, and the papers continued to help raise funds throughout its earliest years on the water. In daily newspapers during the summer and in every annual report, there is a note of gratitude for the support of the press. Every week, the *Boston Evening Transcript* published the contributions received to date. Gifts were even received from other parts of the country: the first donation for the 1895 season was from an otherwise unidentified "Gentleman on the Mississippi River."[10] This was followed by many small and some larger contributions: $2.00 came from seven little girls in Arlington; $100 from Mrs. Thayer of Lancaster; $1.00 from the South Evangelical Sunday School, West Roxbury; $2.25 from the Longfellow Literary Circle, Brockton; $5.00 from a "friend."

People of all sorts, well-to-do and middle class, fashionable society ladies and children, garden clubs and sewing circles, were all attracted to helping the hospital and its little patients. In just a few years, it became one of Boston's most popular charities thanks in large part to the publicity in the newspapers. It was widely referred to as "a beautiful philanthropy."

On August 26, 1897, the *Herald* reported that five hundred people had gathered at Mrs. John Shephard's "palatial residence" making it "the brightest spot on the North Shore last evening." Seated on the enclosed verandas of Mrs. Shephard's house, guests were treated to an evening of *tableaux vivants* and musical selections to benefit the Floating. "Potted palms and golden rod beautified the stage which had been set up to hide the front entrance." "A Western Morning" was the name of one of the tableaux performed by Ms. Ethel Burton, who was later joined by Walter Hitchcock for another performance, "Pygmalion and Galatea." Mrs. Lucia V. Faunce presented vocal selections, and a recitation and the Mozart Quartet of Boston played.

The *Herald* reported that the ladies wore "charming costumes," while the men were resplendent in full evening

The Boston Herald's report on a charity party at the house of Mrs. John Shephard. August 26, 1897.

FOR THE FLOATING HOSPITAL.

A Fine Entertainment Adds Materially to the Fund.

Mrs. John Shepard Throws Open Her Palatial Residence at Beach Bluff for Charity's Sake—North Shore Society Folk Bestow Liberal Patronage—Music and Tableaux.

Mrs. John Shepard's palatial residence on Atlantic avenue, Beach Bluff, was the brightest spot on the North Shore last evening, the occasion being an entertainment given for the benefit of the Floating Hospital fund. The verandas were inclosed and brilliantly illuminated with vari-colored electric lights, the large hall and parlors were arranged to seat the large audience present, and at one end of the hall a stage was arranged, completely hiding the front entrance. Potted plants and golden rod beautified the stage and spacious parlors.

At 7:30 o'clock the guests began to arrive. Handsome turnouts brought many of the smart set, the ladies being attired in charming costumes, and the men in full evening dress.

dress. The *Herald* did not reveal how much money was raised, but all the proceeds of the gala evening went to the hospital.

This sort of fundraising continued as long as the Floating was on the water. In response to a query about her memories of the Floating, Mrs. Joan G. Magary of Woodbury, Connecticut, wrote that when she and her sister were children in the 1920s, they held a magic lantern show in a tent in her family's backyard. Admission was two cents. Those who attended saw a stereopticon slide show featuring the Grand Canyon, the Rockies, and Yellowstone National Park. Lemonade was also for sale, and by the end of the summer, the sisters had collected $8.12 for the Floating.

In 1896, the Floating became a department of Hale's Ten Times One Society, which had been involved in the hospital's development from the beginning. Reverend Tobey was named chairman of The Boston Floating Hospital Committee, and Mr. Roger E. Tileston was treasurer. This arrangement was of financial benefit to the hospital because the fundraising was consolidated within the Ten Times One Society.

During the second year, Boston merchants and businessmen donated many of the items the hospital needed, including crackers, sugar, cocoa, napkins, and enough paper bags for the season. Wollaston florist Mr. Robert Patterson even donated flowers, and others gave the Floating generous discounts. Organizations like the Books and Basket Club and the Helping Hand of Grace Church provided infant clothing, bedding, picture books, and toys. In one of the first seasons on the water, there came a second appeal for more toys. The children on one trip thought they could take the toys home with them, and the volunteers did not have the heart to tell them otherwise.

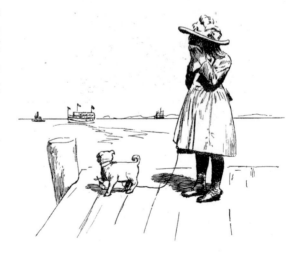

A drawing from the 1902 Annual Report titled "Thou art so near and yet so far."

The newspapers continued to promote the hospital with stories studded with touching anecdotes about the "precious cargo." The *Herald* featured a colored drawing of the hospital that was later used as a fundraising pamphlet printed on paper donated by the St. Botolph's press. The sometimes overly dramatized stories did their work. The Floating had captured the city's imagination. There was something romantic and appealing about the little barge as it floated in the harbor; its high visibility and the nature of its mission made it a popular cause.

AN EXPERIMENTAL SUCCESS! NEW NEEDS ARISE

By the second year of operation, it had become clear to the Floating's administrators that they needed to buy the *Clifford*. Owning the boat would make the arduous process of outfitting the barge before each trip unnecessary. In addition, the image of a boat that was used for pleasure at night and as a hospital by day did not reflect their intention to make the Floating into a permanent institution serving sick children. The second annual report included a strong plea for funds so that "we could make more trips each summer (on a boat) that could be fitted up for the sole use of the hospital." The goal was five trips weekly for nine weeks during the hottest part of the summer the next year. The increase in the number of trips was necessary because the children of the poor continued to get sick during the summer months at an alarming rate.

During the season of 1895, each ward on the barge was designated for the care of a particular sort of patient: the older children or those not so gravely ill were on the upper deck, average cases in the middle, and the more serious cases in the "sick ward." Each ward had its own staff of doctors and nurses. As soon as the barge left the dock, doctors and nurses began their rounds. Sick children were fed at 10:30 in the morning and at 1:15 and 3:15 in the afternoon. Infants were fed more often. At noon, the mothers and all the well children were given lunch. Meals were purposely kept simple [11] so that people would not come aboard just for the food. A typical lunch consisted of corned beef and mutton with cheese and coffee, cocoa, and milk. Later, the Floating's chowder gained a reputation for excellence.

During one of the trips, a young violinist named Frank Spolidoro [12] was photographed by a newspaper cameraman while playing his fiddle for a tiny African-American child sitting at his feet. Little Arthur Simpson was

Admission ticket and instructions for the Floating's third season, the summer of 1896.

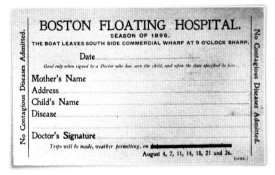

suffering from a severe cough, the papers reported. Spolidoro went along on several trips to entertain the passengers and do small chores for the nurses. The picture, often reprinted in Floating Hospital fundraising documents in subsequent years, demonstrates an important fact: the Floating did not discriminate. Patients of all races and creeds were welcomed on board as were the children of recent immigrants, who were also often discriminated against by other institutions. [13] Indeed, the tickets for the Floating stated that sick children under the age of six, "without distinction of creed, color or nationality," were welcome on board. And this credo was repeated often in its publications and fundraising appeals.

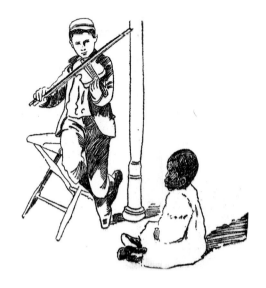

"Little Frank Spolidoro, who goes on every trip with this fiddle to make a few pennies and help in carrying cups, made sweet music."—The Babies' Outing, 1895

By 1897 there was enough money on hand to permit the board to purchase the *Clifford* for five thousand dollars. On June 23, 1897, a preliminary trip was arranged for the members of The Monday Evening Club on the newly refurbished boat. Only forty ailing children and their mothers were aboard as the two hundred fifty members of the club were shown the new bathrooms where sea water baths were available as well as a new ward for serious cases on the lower level. White-painted iron cots donated during the previous winter replaced almost all the hammocks.

Also by 1897, there were seven or eight physicians on board for each trip, and Ms. L.A. Wilber was made the Superintendent of Nurses, a job she would hold for many years. Doctors examined the children when they came on board and placed the patients under the nurses' care. Those day patients who needed more care were given tickets for a return visit. Bedside histories were now routine, and doctors and nurses visited most of the sickest children in their homes for follow up. This home care service greatly enlarged the scope of the hospital by providing continuity of care for the patients. The on-shore hospital that was to be established in 1916 had its origins in these early visits and in the recognition on the part of the doctors that keeping the child well required periodic home visits. Although the first Visiting Nurse Association had been established in the Boston Dispensary in 1886, the idea of nurses visiting patients in their homes was still rather progressive.

In 1897, two children who were too sick to go home at the end of the day were kept on the boat while it went out into the harbor at night. The Floating

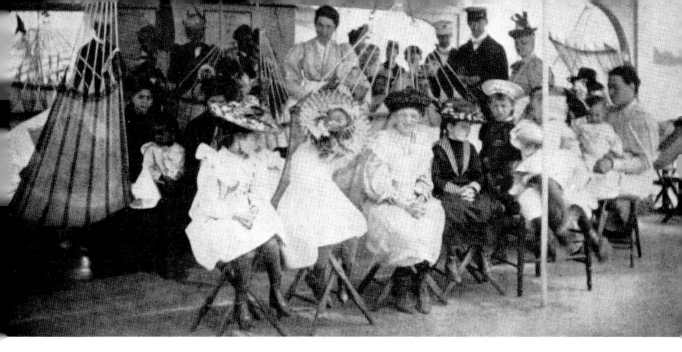

The open air ward on the Clifford. Taken in 1896.

had purchased a special anchor to make this possible, and from then on, the hospital kept its sickest patients on board until they recovered. With the inauguration of these first "permanent wards," the Floating became a full-fledged hospital, not just an outpatient emergency clinic where children found a day's temporary relief.

The hospital now had two wards, which were able to accommodate thirty of the sickest children, and doctors divided patients into two groups. There were the "day patients," who could be treated during a day's trip with perhaps a return or home visits, and the "permanent patients," the much more seriously ill babies who were kept on board as long as needed. The permanent patients' parents had access to them whenever the boat was at the dock. While they could also continue to accompany their children on trips, most parents had other children at home so they could not spend every day on board. The hospital's accessibility was considered a "conspicuous advantage" by the staff. Parents felt comfortable leaving the children in the

Awaiting a doctor's notes, from the 1897 season.

A call for nurse volunteers before the 1897 season. April 26, 1897.

— THE —

BOSTON FLOATING HOSPITAL.

Ward   Trip   Date

Name   Age

DIAGNOSIS.

Diet   B

Boston Floating Hospital.

THE FLOATING HOSPITAL COMMITTEE

Desires to express its appreciation of the volunteer services of nurses (chiefly graduates) in the past, and again appeals to those formerly so connected with the Hospital and to other nurses for help during the coming season.

Trips will be made four times weekly during July and August of this year.

Any nurse wishing to make one or more trips at any time when disengaged during these months will kindly send her name and address to the undersigned as soon as convenient.

SAMUEL BRECK, M. D., *Medical Director.*

April 26, '97.   172 Commonwealth Avenue.

hospital's care because they were encouraged to come on board any time the boat was docked. They did this willingly because they had shared in the child's care from the start and they knew the staff, especially the nurses, and trusted them.

Patients could also be brought onto the Floating at 4:00 p.m. when it arrived at Commercial Wharf in the North End at the end of a day's trip, or any time from 4:30 p.m. to 8:30 a.m. at Pickert's Wharf in East Boston. The daily trips began at Commercial Wharf between 8:30 and 9:00 a.m. A supervising physician was on board around the clock to take care of these very sick infants.

CHANGING ATTITUDES TOWARD POOR MOTHERS

If the attitude of parents had changed toward the hospital, that is because the hospital's treatment of parents had changed as well. In those days, most hospitals still purposely prevented parents from visiting their children—or at least discouraged them from doing so. Visiting hours were deliberately set during the working weekday, and there were no visiting hours on weekends. Healthy children were not permitted in the hospital. These stringent rules made it virtually impossible for parents to find the time to see their sick children. By contrast, and with a revolutionary policy, the Floating routinely provided free access to parents of all patients.

The doctors who served on the Floating in the early days came from the Boston Dispensary, which was established in 1796 as the first permanent medical facility in New England. In 1856, the Boston Dispensary abolished the prevailing system that allowed wealthy subscribers, by dint of their support, to indicate who was to be treated. At the Boston Dispensary, physicians made the decisions, and, for a very low annual fee, patients received prepaid medical care. It could be said that the Dispensary was an early model of a Health Maintenance Organization.

Doctors who joined the Floating brought this enlightened culture with them. The Floating's radical approach to how parents were treated seemed to have a generally positive effect on the enterprise and the care of the patients. The annual reports mention that cases of parents interfering with the hospital's care and discipline of the children were "almost unheard of." The directors could see no reason to regret their "very liberal rules in this respect. Parents have frequently expressed their appreciation to the nurses and doctors for what was done."[14]

BOSTON PRESS
AND THE FLOATING

An article in the *Boston Herald* described a typical Sunday on board:[3]

"The boat lay all day at Pickert's Wharf, East Boston. The first thing one notices is the Sabbath-like stillness on board. There is no more noise than in any household. The church bells are heard in the distance, but are almost unnoticed, for on the Hospital work and worship are synonymous ... Dr. R. W. Hastings is the resident physician, and limited quarters are all he can have in this crowded boat, for a sleeping-room and for the clerical work that is necessary ... The Sunday force of nurses and medical assistants is on duty from 7:15 a.m. until 8 p.m. excepting those who have time off. All their meals are taken on board the boat. When the day nurses begin their work they find the patients partly prepared for the day by the night nurses. At 7:30 comes their first feeding and it is no slight task to care for 57 sick babies, some of them very ill indeed, some very feeble from illness and others convalescent and ready to be discharged.

"After this all the patients are bathed if they are well enough, then the wards are put in order for the visiting physicians, who come over from the city to see each patient, and who spend an hour or two on board. The house doctors have had their breakfast and are now ready for their duty. At 9:30 comes the next feeding, the food coming in bottles fresh from the food laboratory on the lower deck. Every minute of the time is employed. The babies are changed frequently and their bedding renewed. On Sunday nearly 1,000 napkins [diapers] are used. On week days when the day patients are on board, the number is 1500, taking 1400 yards of gauze and 100 pounds of absorbent cotton-waste. They are destroyed after being used. On week days many of the mothers on board assist in making them.

"Dinner is served from 12 Noon to 1:30 on Sundays and supper from five to six o'clock. At eight the night force reports for duty. It consists of two senior house doctors, a night matron, two to four nurses in each ward, the night watchman, engineer, assistant in the food laboratory, scrub woman, stewardess, three sailors. The resident physician is always on board. All the day staff sleep on shore. A meal is served to the night force at 12 o'clock. The patients are not fed as often during the night, but are encouraged to sleep. The lights are shaded, and the boat is as quiet as possible. Occasionally the silence is punctured by the sharp ring of the telephone bell. Some anxious mother cannot sleep and has called from the nearest drug-store at midnight to find our how her darling is passing the night, for to such watchers morning seems so long in coming, and it does not always bring welcome news.

"Another feature of Sunday is visits by physicians and students and they are always welcome as Sunday being a quiet day they have better opportunities to study the work. Yesterday a surgeon of the United States navy inspected the Hospital. This season Dr. Hastings has been sending reply postal cards to the physicians who have sent patients to the boat, offering to send them reports of the cases at intervals if they so desire. This courtesy is much appreciated and shows the wish of the Hospital to co-operate with different doctors.

"When it is a bright, warm Sunday the boat goes out into the harbor, that the patients may have the benefit of the fresh cool air. Parents wishing to see their children are told to come to the dock at 3:30 p.m. when the boat returns. But on a wet Sunday she remains at the wharf and they come when they can."

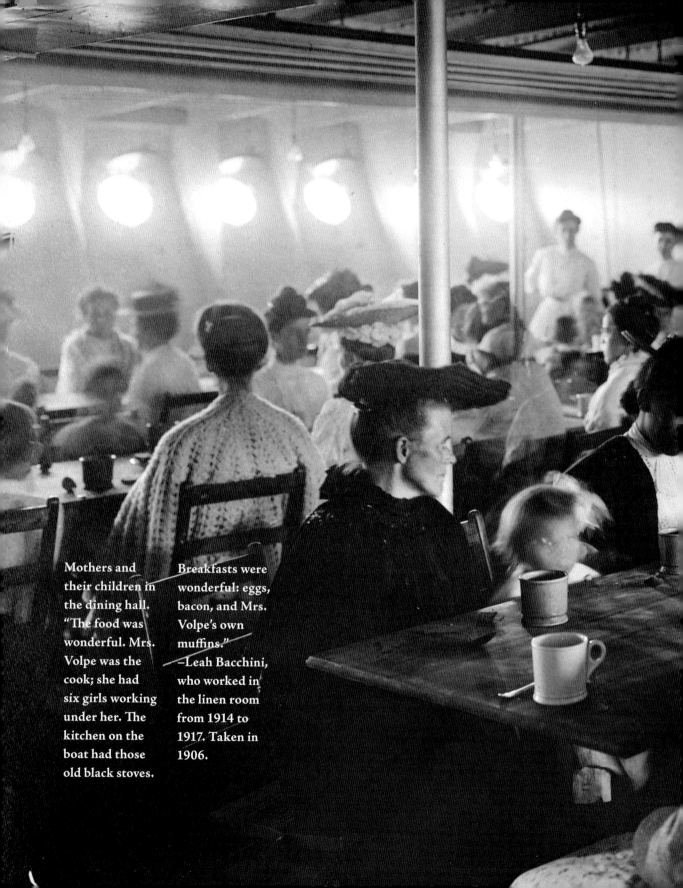

Mothers and their children in the dining hall. "The food was wonderful. Mrs. Volpe was the cook; she had six girls working under her. The kitchen on the boat had those old black stoves. Breakfasts were wonderful: eggs, bacon, and Mrs. Volpe's own muffins."
—Leah Bacchini, who worked in the linen room from 1914 to 1917. Taken in 1906.

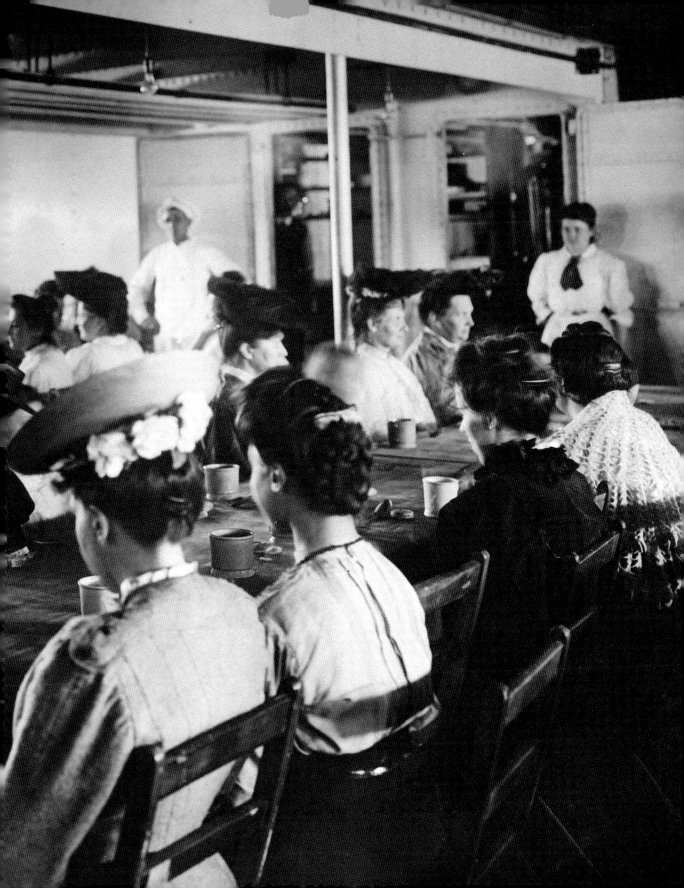

Unlike most of the hospitals of that time, the Floating did not look down on uneducated mothers or blame those immigrant women who did not understand much English and needed help in learning how to take better care of their children.

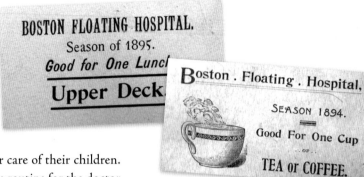

For example, it was part of the routine for the doctor at the gangplank to search the bags mothers brought on board for contraband food. Green apples, sweets, unsanitary milk, and other foods were "fed to the fishes." But this was done in a kindly, gentle, and nonjudgmental manner so that mothers would not consider it a punishment. Wholesome food brought on board was returned to the mothers as they left. The unhealthy food and drink they tried to bring aboard was destroyed after explanations about why this was necessary. Mothers were given vouchers in exchange for their food entitling them and their healthy children to lunch on board, and refreshments were served to them later in the day.

However, mothers were not only permitted to remain on board with their babies—they were, from day one, encouraged to form a partnership with the doctors and nurses overseeing their child's care. The children were treated with compassion, the mothers with dignity. Moreover, by 1896, the Floating recognized that there were often other children in the family who could not be left alone at home, and mothers were allowed to bring one healthy child onto the boat if necessary. The Floating provided a kindergarten for healthy children under the age of six. This daycare facility gave their mothers free time to concentrate on their sick child and provided the healthy youngster with a pleasant excursion at sea.

From the first voyages of the Floating, there were classes to teach mothers how to take better care of their children. These classes became more formalized as the years went by. The mothers were present when the physicians and nurses examined the children, and they were taught how to prepare the formula, how to sterilize bottles, and how to recognize and give early treatment for childhood diseases. The founders of the Floating understood that the mothers were a vital component in the process of healing the children. Educating the mothers was as important as taking care of the babies while they were on the boat. The first annual report explained:

"One of the chief objects aimed at in The Boston Floating Hospital is to place the responsibility for the care of the sick baby upon the mother. While on board The Boston Floating Hospital, a doctor and a nurse look out for its welfare; she is taught what to do for the child between trips and reports each time she returns with it. The experience thus acquired is invaluable." [15]

By 1897, the nurses held more organized and structured mothers' classes on every trip in order to teach "those who have the care of helpless young lives." For sixty-five cents ("prices which bring them within the means of the poorest woman") mothers were able to buy sterilizers and twelve baby bottles. [16] The nurses showed the mothers how to sterilize milk and how to cleanse bottles and nipples. These classes showed them the best way of caring for their babies in their own homes. "Inasmuch as the highest function of any charitable institution is to help people care for themselves, this element of the work may be regarded as a valuable one," the hospital's directors stated. The mothers' classes became a landmark innovation. While other charitable hospitals were doing their best to keep mothers separate from the care of their own children, the Floating was taking steps to create partnerships with families in order to provide the best care possible for the children who needed it most.

Here are the instructions doctors provided to mothers so that they could take the lessons they learned on the ship home to their families: [17]

To Sterilize Milk

Take a Mason Jar or other large-mouthed bottle. Have it perfectly clean, fill it two-third full of milk, then put a piece of cotton batting over the mouth, tying it on with a clean white cord or tape. Place in a kettle on a block of wood or some straw; then pour in warm water, till it comes up to the milk; set on top of, or in the stove if fire is slow. Put the cover tightly on the kettle when the water boils, remove from the fire, keeping it covered close. Let it stand in the kettle on the back of stove 40 minutes. Then take from kettle keeping the cotton batting over the mouth. When needed, pour into infant's bottle covering the jar with the cotton batting. Put the nursing bottle in water hot enough to warm. To each feeding add 2 table-spoonfuls of Lime Water. It is best to sterilize twice a day during the hot weather. Keep milk in a cool place out of the sun.

To Cleanse Bottles

Rinse in cold water, wash in hot soap suds, scald and when cool, fill with water into which you have put a pinch of soda.

To Cleanse Nipples

Rinse in cold water, turn wrong side out, wash in soda and water, put in cold water on stove in a dish and boil ten minutes, remove and put in clean cup of cold water which has a little soda in it. Use no tin ware about a child's food. Keep milk, water, gruel, etc. in china pitcher or glass jar.

There were special instructions also for the feeding of small children. To contemporary mothers, these will sound quaint and even silly, but for the mothers of that time they provided valuable guidelines about nutrition. Proper food was an essential aspect of the infants' care and was in large measure the fundamental treatment for their intestinal disorders. By the turn of the twentieth century, when the food laboratory had been established on board, twenty different kinds of foods or combinations of foods were used to prepare the formula for the infants on the Floating Hospital.

In the early days, instructions given to the mothers of children over one year of age were precise:

DIET DIRECTIONS FOR CHILDREN OVER
ONE YEAR OLD

The less solid food given before a child is a year old the better. After this age what milk the child takes should be sterilized the same as before but the PLAIN MILK should be used. LITTLE BY LITTLE solid food should be added to the diet, beginning with one meal of such food a day, then two, then three if the food suits. If any vomiting or diarrhea results, return to liquids until these symptoms stop. The child should be fed at REGULAR TIMES and not be allowed to eat at any other times. The eating of fruit, crackers, candy, pastry, etc., between meals is the cause of a great deal of sickness.

The first solid to give the baby is white bread twenty-four hours old, the soft part, and from this gradually on to boiled rice, farina, cerealine, fine hominy oat meal (not more than two or three times a week), yolk of a dropped egg on toast and corn starch pudding. The child should still have plenty of milk. No meat should be allowed until the child is two

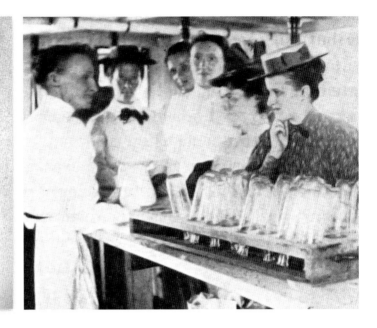

Helpful instructions for mothers from The Floating Hospital.

Mother's learn how to sterilize bottles. Taken in 1898.

years of age. Fish like cod or haddock, may be eaten, also baked or boiled potato. Plain water crackers are good but sweet crackers or soda crackers are not at all so. Broths from which the fat has been removed are good. Cooked fruits such as baked apples (not the skin) and stewed prunes may be given.

The child must not have anything fried or greasy, salt meat (ham, bacon, etc.) beans, cabbage, hard boiled or fried eggs, candy, pastry, apples, bananas, berries, green vegetables, pork, nuts, cake or cheese.

These classes that educated mothers on how best to care for their children may seem commonplace today, but they were nothing short of revolutionary at the time. Indeed, the classes were only the first of many innovations that made the Floating a pioneer in patient care. It took several decades after those initial voyages before the hospital realized its full potential, but from the launching of its very first trip, it was engaged in a remarkable experiment in the provision of health care. Its manner of serving its patients differed in important ways from how the hospitals of that time functioned.

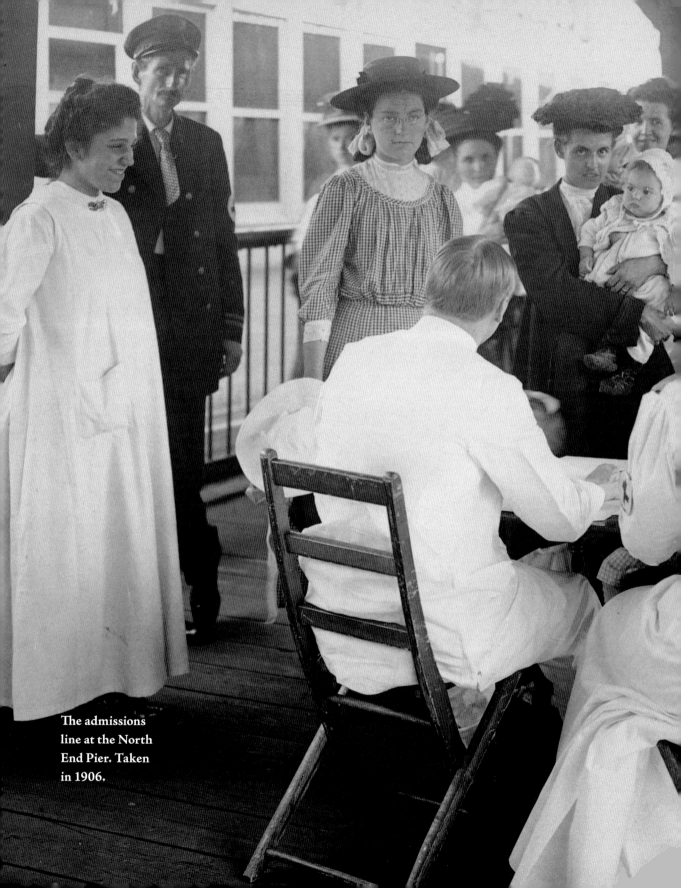

The admissions
line at the North
End Pier. Taken
in 1906.

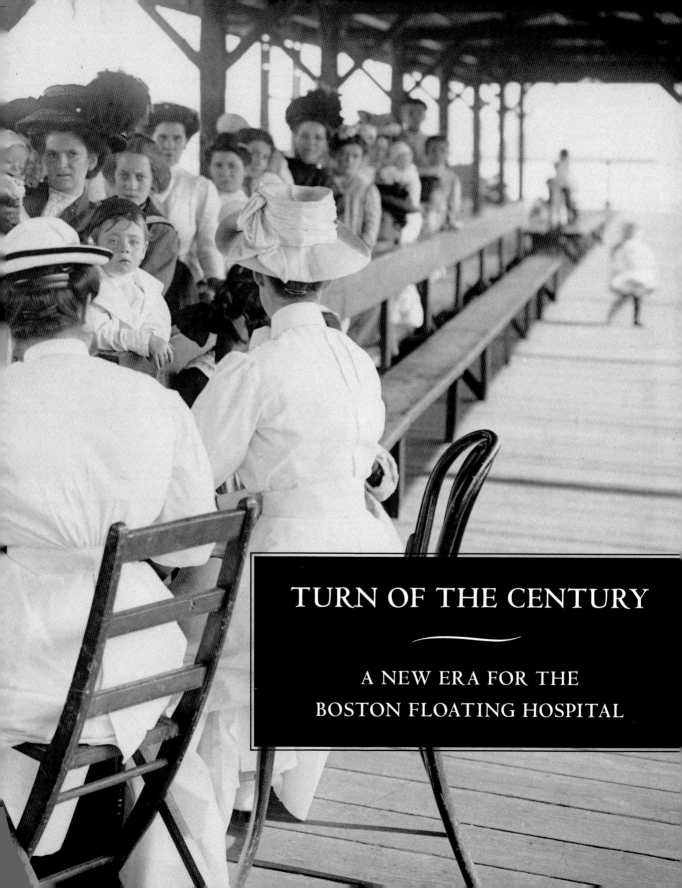

TURN OF THE CENTURY

A NEW ERA FOR THE
BOSTON FLOATING HOSPITAL

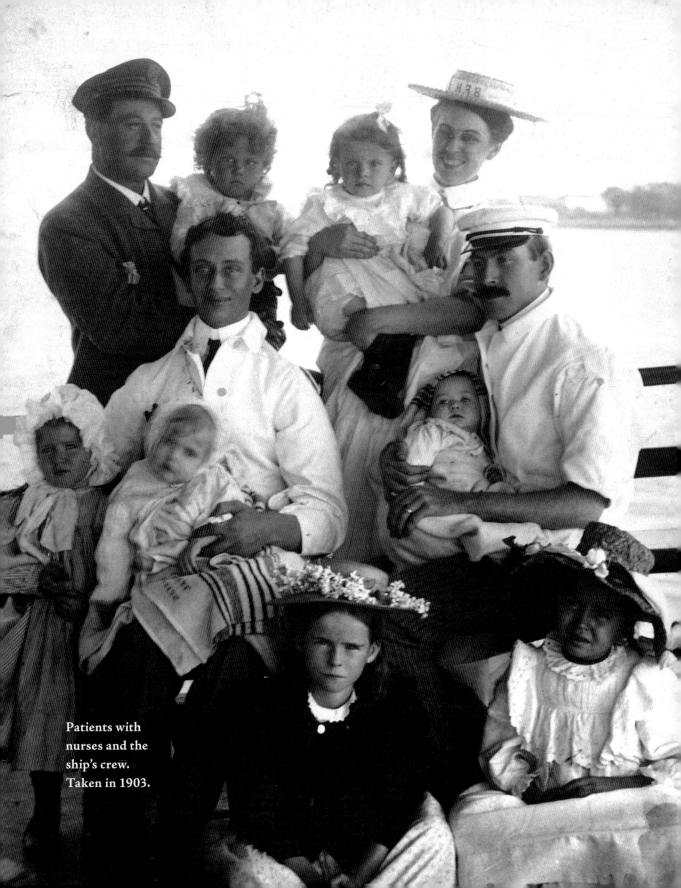

Patients with
nurses and the
ship's crew.
Taken in 1903.

TURN OF THE CENTURY
A NEW ERA FOR THE BOSTON FLOATING HOSPITAL

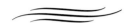

The early 1900s was a time of change for The Boston Floating Hospital. The Floating had been in existence only six years but had already earned a national reputation as the only place in the country where pediatric summer diseases could be studied. Physicians and nurses came from all over the country to serve on board. The clinical area had been enlarged, and a similar expansion of the hospital's laboratory was the logical next step. A physiological laboratory equipped with a microscopy unit was the goal.

In truth, the Floating had just about outgrown the *Clifford* by 1900. It had enlarged its original mandate and no longer confined itself to only the diseases of early childhood; doctors were now treating older children as well. As a result of this expansion of services, patients flocked to the ship in droves.

The purchase of a new boat became a necessity; this new boat, along with advances in children's medicine, set the stage for the hospital's innovative and significant contributions to pediatrics for decades to come.

BUYING A NEW SHIP
Overflowing with Children and Raising Funds for the New Boat

The summer of 1905 was unusually hot, resulting in a record number of patients, particularly in July. But more children than ever before had to be turned away, heightening the expectations for a larger vessel. Luckily, the new boat was no longer just a distant dream. It was "assured for next season," marking the culmination of eleven years of diligent work. Details of the plans for the new boat were made public in the annual report for 1905.[1]

Refusing patients must have been the most difficult thing the staff did. Every day the *Clifford* was filled to capacity, and the permanent wards were full early in the season. In a particularly vivid report[2] of this problem, Robert W. Hastings, the resident physician, stated that in 1904, 279 patients had to be turned away. In 1902 they turned far more away, but 1903 saw a slight dip to 207 surplus patients. No cause for rejoicing here, Dr. Hastings hastened to add, since there were more beds only because more very sick babies were admitted and more of them died, freeing up beds for other children. But, he added, the visiting physicians "moved patients along more rapidly" toward recovery too.

Due to their growing needs, the trustees had inaugurated a concerted effort beginning in 1901 to raise the funds for a boat that could accommodate at least one hundred permanent patients and one hundred day patients,

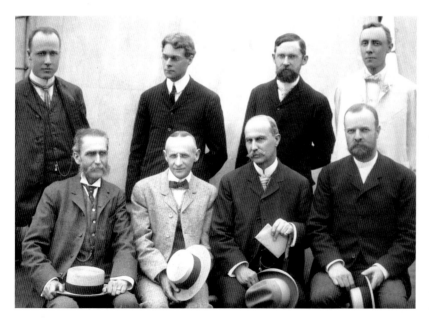

Standing from left to right: Herbert Winslow Hill, Director Bacteriological Laboratory, Boston Board of Health; Dr. Arthur I. Kendall, Rockefeller Fellow, Boston Floating Hospital; Dr. William Fay, Visiting Staff, Boston Floating Hospital; Dr. Robert W. Hastings, Resident Physician, Boston Floating Hospital. Sitting from left to right: Rufus B. Tobey, Chairman, Board of Managers, Boston Floating Hospital; Dr. Simon Flexner, University of Pennsylvania; Dr. Samuel H. Durgin, Chairman of the Board of Health; Dr. Samuel Breck, Chief of Visiting Staff, Boston Floating Hospital. Date unknown.

designed to meet the hospital's own specifications. It would take five years before this vision would become a reality.

Because the hospital did not charge its patients, it had to find ways to expand contributions to fund the purchase of a new boat. It established named days and nights, so that a patron could dedicate a day or night on the ship to a particular person. As a modest attempt to raise more funds, the price of named days was raised from one hundred dollars to one hundred fifty dollars, named nights cost one hundred dollars, and named beds cost two hundred fifty dollars. Three grades of membership in The Boston Floating Hospital Corporation were now available: First, persons paying one hundred dollars or more and requesting membership; Second, persons paying ten dollars for annual membership; Third, an associate membership for children paying one dollar or more and requesting annual membership.[3]

On September 23, 1901, after the end of that year's hospital season, the Lend-a-Hand-Society (the Ten Times One Society) transferred all its rights in the Floating, which it had held since May 1896, to a corporation that was established to manage the newly expanded institution. The Boston Floating Hospital Corporation's first meeting was held on November 4, 1901, and elected Reverend Rufus Babcock Tobey as chairman, S. Homer Woodbridge as vice chairman, and Charles G. Farwell as treasurer and business manager.[4] The newly constituted board announced its goal to launch a new boat in June 1903 in time for that summer's season.

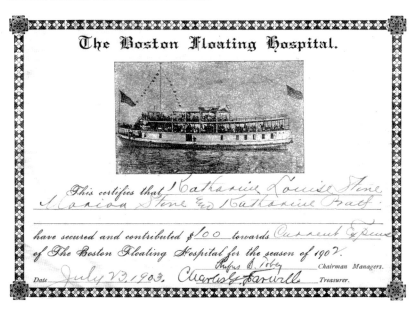

Certificate for a $100 donation during the 1903 season.

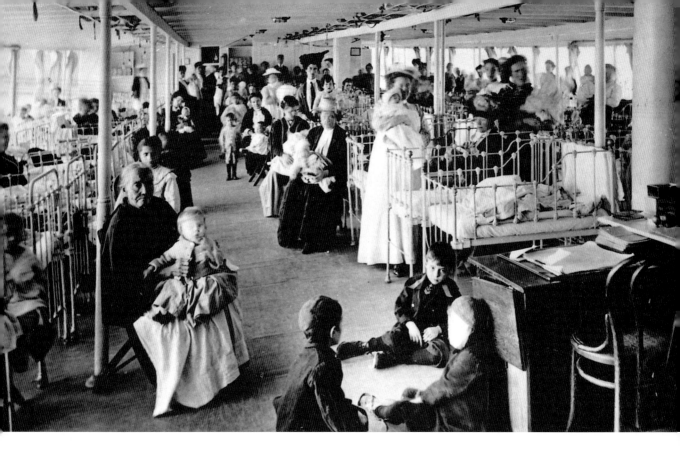

Day patients' open ward deck. Taken in 1909.

The summer of 1902 was unseasonably cool, and this resulted in a fundraising disaster, as the public mistakenly thought that the boat was not needed as badly in cool weather. Only about one-fifth of the probable cost of the new boat had been raised. In the 1902 annual report, the board of directors hinted darkly that the Floating might have to cancel a season's work if they didn't raise at least fifty thousand dollars by the following year. "The present boat will not answer our purpose after another season and we face the possibility of being compelled to omit a season's work if by August 1, 1903 we do not have construction funds sufficiently large to justify us in giving a contract for the new boat."[5]

Because of the drop in contributions, the directors used a statement by Dr. Simon Flexner to strengthen their appeal for the New Boat Fund. During his visit to the Floating, he observed, "Both permanent and transient wards are very crowded and the work of the doctors as well as the improvement of many of the patients is greatly retarded by lack of space. Boston people ought to redouble their charitable efforts, and contribute enough money for another boat. It is a noble work, and worthy of the attention of everybody."[6] In spite of this and other equally eloquent pleas from the board of directors, the prospects for launching a new home for the Floating were dim as the 1904 season began.

The frugal and prudent directors expressed their disappointment as well as their management philosophy in this way:

"True economy is to get all out of a thing that one can and when it was found that, with necessary repairs there was one more year of service in the Boston Floating Hospital, it seemed to the managers unwise to build the new one, much as it is needed. The arguments for the new boat are as cogent now as they ever have been, but the money for it is not yet available. If the public is disappointed, the managers are no less so; but we shall be compelled to conduct our work in the season of 1905 as in previous years. A purpose to keep free from debt is commendable at any time and everywhere, and it surely is so in the case of the Floating Hospital."[7]

The directors predicted that in future summers, no matter what the weather, but particularly during heat waves, they would soon be overwhelmed unless contributions to build a new boat were received.

The chairman of the visiting staff, Dr. Samuel Breck, made a heartfelt appeal to the contributors: "The writer almost feels his report to have received a mortal blow, so keen is his disappointment. It was expected that a new boat would be ready equipped for next season." He lamented the lack of funds. He estimated it would cost sixty-five to seventy-five thousand dollars to build the boat that has been planned "entirely satisfactory in its appointments, fully equipped and adapted for one hundred permanent patients and two hundred out-patients."[8]

PLANS FOR THE SHIP

The board was very clear that they should build nothing less than the most well-equipped boat. They were not going to compromise on this even though the costs were high. The Floating was now considered a model for hospitals that might be contemplating a similar project. "It is our duty ... to give not only those immediately about us but to all who may profit by it the benefit of our now considerable experience in this peculiar work. Therefore, an inadequate boat would not only be unserviceable for our immediate uses but would be a disgrace to all concerned."[9]

By 1904, three-fifths of the money had been raised. Dr. Breck argued that it would be better to wait for the rest rather than enter a "mortgage nightmare."

The Floating should build the new boat with a clear conscience, a boat that would "present our givers, our community and the profession at large" with a hospital that they could proudly display to others. Planning and fundraising continued in tandem.

It had been decided that the hull would be made of steel because of its durability, cleanliness, and safety. It would make the boat practically unsinkable. The hull was to be divided into seven watertight compartments in order to provide much more room for patients than the *Clifford* had. The boat's dimensions were to be 170 feet by 46.5 feet, purposely broad for added stability. The *Clifford* had to be towed into the harbor, but the new boat would be constructed so that machinery for self-propulsion—twin engines—could be installed in the future.

There were to be four decks. The one in the hull or lower deck would provide ample room for two large steam boilers with the necessary pumps for supplying hot and cold water to all parts of the boat. The pumps would also provide water in case of fire and could be used to eject water from the hold. Room was to be set aside for the refrigerating and ventilating apparatus and the "machinery for self propulsion," which were to be installed as soon as the hospital had the necessary funds.

A large, well-lighted, and ventilated dining room for the mothers and their healthy children was to be situated on the lower deck. The room would do double duty as a lecture room since it would be comparatively free from noise. The lower deck would also house the mortuary and autopsy room.

The dining room for the house officers and nurses was to be on the main deck. Commodious quarters, well-lighted and ventilated, were to be provided on this deck for the food laboratory. This area was to be arranged "with a due sense of its great importance." In addition, an extra ward to be used only in case of emergency was set up. The clinical laboratory and various rooms and offices were to be on the main deck.

The main hospital deck would consist of six large wards with one hundred beds for permanent patients. The four central wards were to be reserved for the sickest patients, and each was constructed so that it could be fumigated without affecting the adjoining wards, which were to be cooled and ventilated by the atmospheric plant machinery.[10]

Convalescents were to be kept in the bow of the boat because it was admirably adapted for that purpose. The out-of-doors ward in the stern was expected to be of great value in many cases, especially chronic disease, because it was sheltered from high winds and could be closed in if necessary. The operating room was also to be on this deck.

The top deck was to accommodate one hundred fifty to two hundred day patients. On the old boat, this deck was open to the elements so that in bad weather the patients would have to be taken below. But the new deck was well-sheltered, which would make it much more useful. An examination and treatment room was to be on the top deck as were abundant toilet and bath facilities. The bow room was set apart for the kindergarten, for the guests, and as a resting room for the nurses. Quarters for the resident physician and the house officers were to be in the stern. A room for the visiting staff would include a library in the near future.

In the plans for the superstructure, the need to ensure against the hazard of a fire on board received "first consideration," and there was a great deal of discussion about this. It was suggested that sheet metal be used for partitions. The fire-proofing of wood was also under consideration, but in the end it was decided "the best protection of the boat against fire, aside from her steel hull,

Check-in time for mothers and babies before coming on board the ship. Taken in 1906.

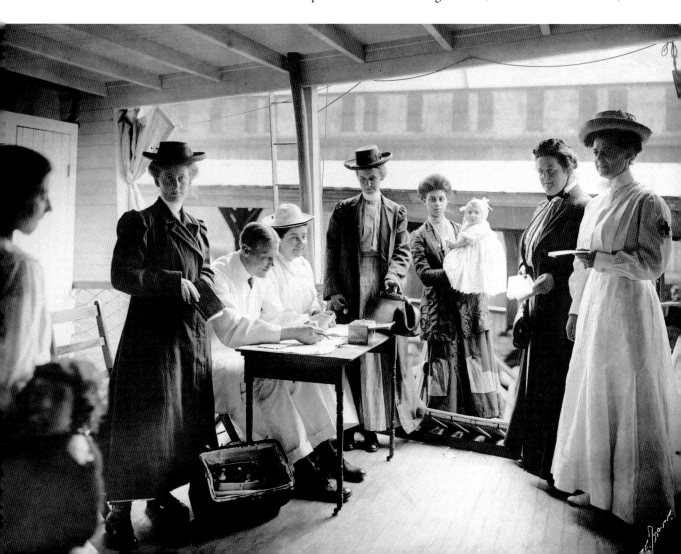

is an efficient fire apparatus." Daily fire drills were part of the hospital's routine on the new ship. The following eyewitness account comes from the January 1917 issue of *The Nurse: The Journal of Pediatric Knowledge*: "The medical and nursing staff were assigned fixed stations in lifeboats in case of fire. Periodically, at a blast from the steam whistle, the lifeboats were lowered into the water and nurses and doctors practiced emergency drills using bundles of cloth to simulate the babies who were passed from the deck into the lifeboats. The entire drill took only two minutes."[11]

The boat was built and put into service at a cost of $174,000. This money came from contributions and an issue of 5 percent bonds in the amount of $74,000. Several years later, an annual report stated that $52,000 of these bonds had been retired "without appeal to our contributors of the past six years. These bonds mature in April, 1913 and contributions to this amount are asked for in addition to those for current needs."[12]

1906 AND THE NEW BOAT

When the 1906 season opened, the new and eagerly awaited boat was still not quite ready. An account of the early days of that season on the old boat and the maiden voyage of the beautiful new boat in August was written by one of the Floating's nurses, Ms. Josephine Halberstadt.[13]

"The season of 1906 was to be an eventful one in the history of the Boston Floating Hospital. The new boat was to be in commission, and although there was some delay on account of a steel strike during the winter, it was hoped that it would be possible to start the season on the new boat, for which we had waited so long and patiently. But the date of its completion could not be definitely determined, and little patients waiting to be admitted made it necessary to start the season on the old hospital boat, so the first trip was made July 11.

"From the beginning the season promised to be a busy one and although there was some disappointment when it was learned that the new boat could not be ready for some days, both the house staff and the nurses proved their willingness to help in every possible way, and showed the usual interest in their work—which at first seems hard on account of its newness. The work is very different in comparison with usual hospital work, for the patients are very sick babies, most of them under two years of age … The spirit of congeniality is one of the Boston Floating Hospital features. Nurses from almost every state meet as absolute strangers and are here offered an opportunity to give full scope to that broadness which nurses as a rule acquire and in a very short time working unitedly (sic) in this labor of love a general feeling of good-fellowship is established …

"August 14 was to be 'moving day,' for the new boat was now ready for occupancy. The *Clifford*, which had served as a hospital for twelve years was to be deserted and although we were indeed grateful for the beautiful new boat, we could not help feeling somewhat sad to leave the old one with which we associated so many hours, both arduous and pleasant. The packing was done during the day and the babies were given numbers designating the ward and bed to which they would be transferred. Everything was put in readiness so that when Doctor Hastings' order came to move there would be as little confusion as possible.

"The *Clifford* made its last trip down the harbor on this day returning rather earlier than usual. At 3 p.m. when nearing East Boston, we saw

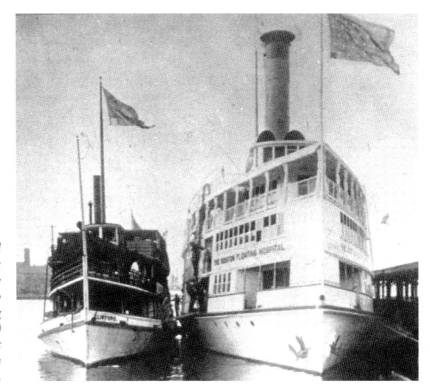

Boston Floating Hospital patients and equipment were moved from the Clifford (on the left) to the New Boston Floating Hospital ship (on the right) while both were docked at the North End Pier. Taken August 14, 1906.

the new Boston Floating Hospital leaving the Atlantic Works and being towed over to North End Pier, which was to be its new abiding place. No doubt we all gave a silent cheer, for she presented a beautiful spectacle indeed in her snowy white robe and decoration of flags. The *Clifford* was towed alongside and when Dr. Hastings said 'go ahead,' in less than one hour every patient was in its new home and also many new ones who had been waiting to be admitted for there were not beds, nor room enough on the *Clifford* to supply the demand, especially during August, when the weather was very oppressive.

"In a few days all the available beds found occupants and even then, with all these extra beds for permanent patients there were not enough to meet the demand and it became necessary to form a permanent ward on the out-patient deck. This ward contained thirty patients, making a total of one hundred and thirty permanent patients and many days one hundred day patients in the out-patient department so the new boat was immediately taxed to its utmost capacity, surely proving its urgent need.

"On August 15 (1906) the new Boston Floating Hospital made its initial trip. It was indeed a gala day. Every boat saluted us, many going out of their way to pass us and we were justly proud of our beautiful new vessel, the first and only one ever designed and built for a hospital boat.

"The season closed September 15th, when patients in fair condition were sent to their respective homes and cases where this was not considered advisable were transferred to hospitals. September 17, 18, 19 the new boat was thrown open for public inspection. Visitors were welcomed by Manager (G. Loring) Briggs and some of the physicians and nurses, they in turn conducting parties through the various wards, operating-room, treatment room, pharmacy/laboratories, dining-rooms, kitchen and store rooms. Questions were willingly answered, interesting features pointed out and explanation given concerning the work of the Floating Hospital. There were over 1,300 visitors in these few days, the same including many prominent people of Boston and its vicinity. All seemed very much pleased, some proving their interest in a substantial way and the universal opinion expressed was to the effect that this is a noble work which is carried on so faithfully on this White Ship of Mercy."

The Bath Department of the City of Boston gave the trustees permission to dock the hospital boat at the pier at North End Park. This pleased the trustees, who thought the new berth an "almost ideal-condition as regards to location, fresh air and saving in expense." The pier was promised to the hospital as a permanent home for both summer and winter. [14]

In the 1906 season, the new hospital was still lacking one important component: the engines required to run the boat under her own power. They were not added for "want of time and money," but it was known that this would be remedied soon. Mrs. L. G. Burnham, a widow whose husband had left her a steam yacht named *Pilgrim*, had donated its engines and boilers to the Floating. The 1906 annual report anticipated her gift, and the engines were installed in 1907. [15] The Floating was now able to enter the harbor proudly under its own steam. The familiar white flag with its green crosses flew from the roof of the cabin, and green crosses were painted on the smoke stack. Emblazoned on its sides were the words: The Boston Floating Hospital.

The inadequacies of the old boat had never been more evident than in its final days. And the weather conditions during the new boat's first summer were so severe that there was an increased patient load. To respond to the ever-growing need, the new boat had to be modified almost as soon as it was in service. A section of the day patients' deck was temporarily converted into a permanent ward with the addition of thirty cribs for children too sick to be sent home. This was possible only because the new vessel had a tight roof, canvas side curtains, and "every convenience." By the end of the season, eighty-three patients had been cared for on the deck as permanent patients, receiving a total of 466 days of care, twenty-four hours a day. [16]

The new Floating Hospital proved its worth during its first tour of duty because it demonstrated that, if necessary, the new boat could accommodate more patients simply by making a few changes. That meant that, in an emergency, it could easily accommodate those day patients found to be too sick to be sent home.

By 1905 the practice of allowing prospective hospital donors to come aboard as guests during the trips was seen to be hindering its work. Guests were now restricted to the late afternoon when the boat had docked and the day patients returned home. The Floating was no longer a curiosity; it was a working hospital, and even would-be donors were not allowed to interfere with its work. Dr. Hastings expressed relief in the report for 1906 that, for the first time, he had been free from the "constant observation all day long" of these visitors.

During the first full season on the new boat, the laundry and the refrigerating system were found to need overhauling. A new laundry big enough to handle the three thousand items that the hospital washed each day was

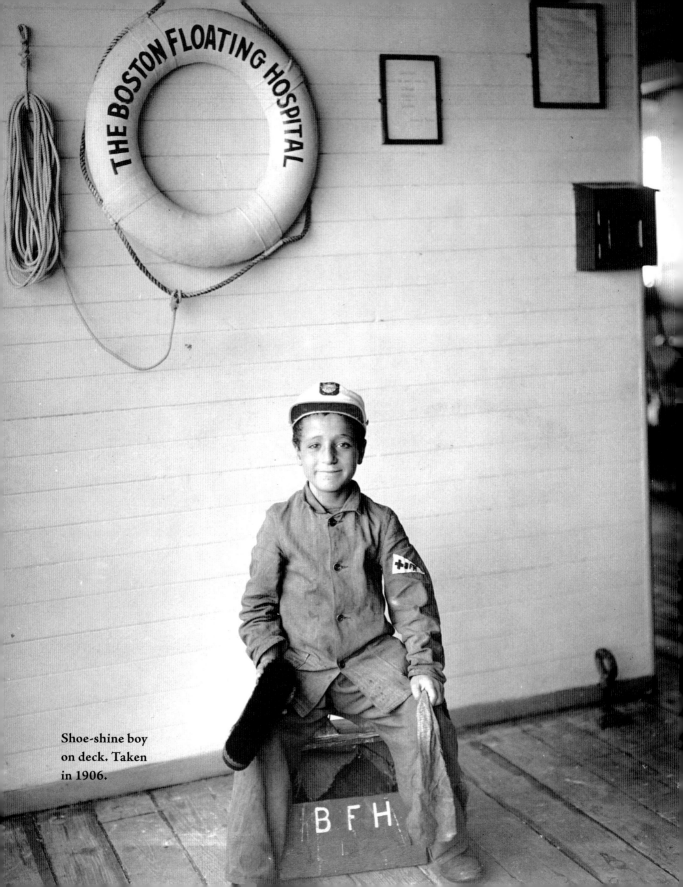

THE BOSTON FLOATING HOSPITAL

Shoe-shine boy
on deck. Taken
in 1906.

B F H

planned for the following year. They also needed a new refrigerating plant that could make enough ice for the circulation of cool, dry, fresh air in the ward every three minutes. [17]

The administration of the hospital was functioning with improved purchasing methods, record keeping, and an inventory of supplies. The linen room, for instance, was now off limits for anyone without an order for supplies from the head nurse. In addition, the personnel needed the time to get accustomed to the new quarters. It could be said that the first summer on the new boat constituted a kind of shakedown cruise for the Floating.

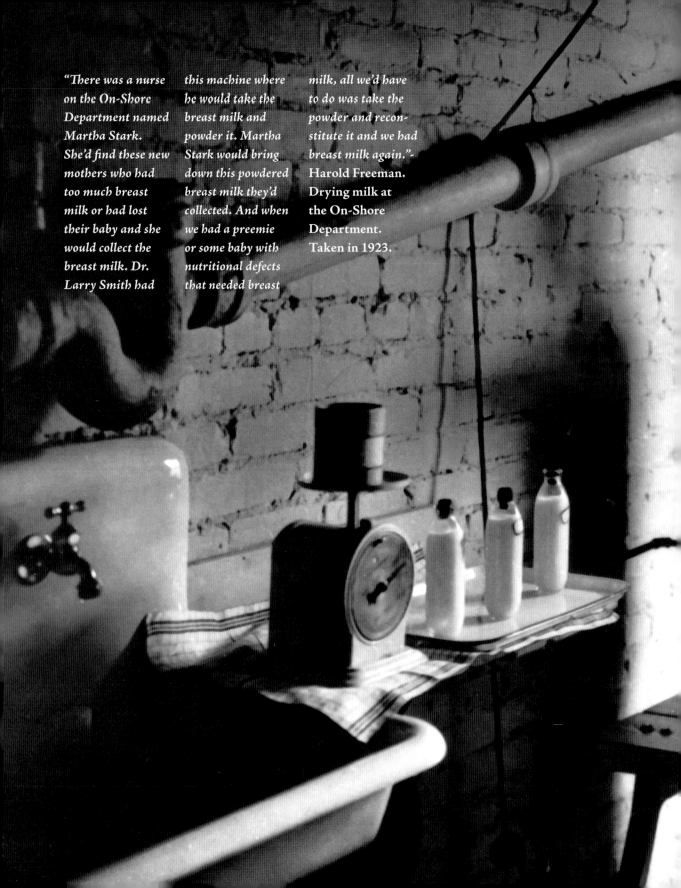

"There was a nurse on the On-Shore Department named Martha Stark. She'd find these new mothers who had too much breast milk or had lost their baby and she would collect the breast milk. Dr. Larry Smith had this machine where he would take the breast milk and powder it. Martha Stark would bring down this powdered breast milk they'd collected. And when we had a preemie or some baby with nutritional defects that needed breast milk, all we'd have to do was take the powder and reconstitute it and we had breast milk again."- Harold Freeman. Drying milk at the On-Shore Department. Taken in 1923.

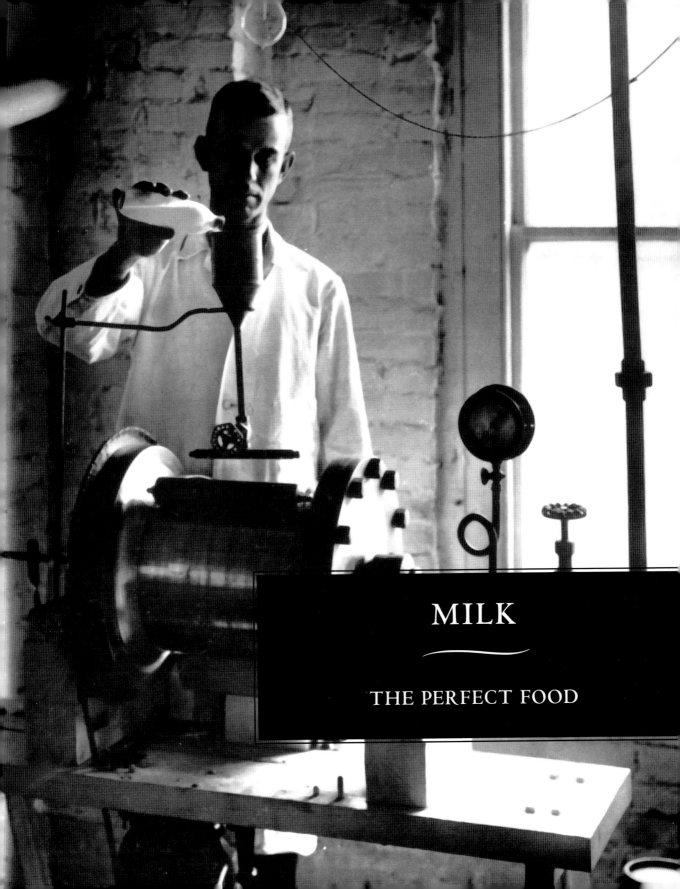

MILK

THE PERFECT FOOD

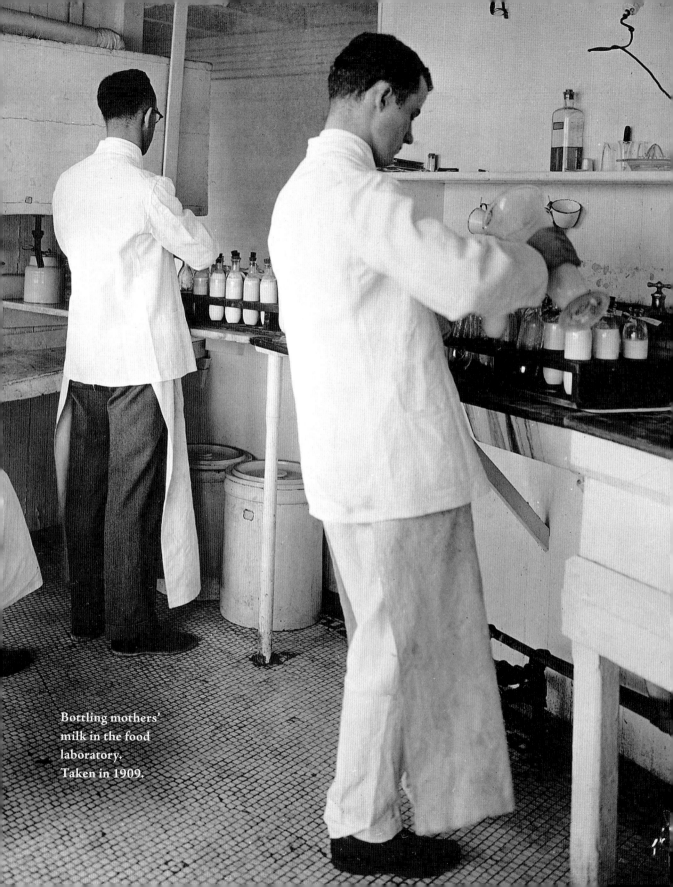

Bottling mothers'
milk in the food
laboratory.
Taken in 1909.

MILK

THE PERFECT FOOD

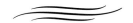

From the nurses who traveled around Boston collecting donated breast milk to the invention of formula, the Floating was always at the forefront of infant nutrition and the advances in the treatment of milk. By the turn of the twentieth century, when the food laboratory had been established on board, doctors were using twenty different kinds of food or combinations of food to prepare formula on the Floating. The hospital's work established how modern-day doctors, nurses, and parents view and use milk and formula.

MILK AT THE BOSTON FLOATING HOSPITAL

By 1909, the Floating was the largest and most important infants' hospital in the United States because it offered doctors an opportunity to study the largest number and variety of the diseases of infants. [1] Several of these studies were subsequently published. "Studies in Intestinal Disturbances in Infants" was reprinted in the *Boston Medical and Surgical Journal*, March 2, 1911, and further papers deriving from the work done by the staff of the Floating in 1911-1912 were published in the same journal in 1913. [2]

Intestinal diseases continued to be alleviated and controlled through modifying the babies' food, and since milk was basic food for young children, the investigators increasingly focused on the role of milk in those illnesses. The Floating was a pioneer in providing formulas made from cows' milk and other ingredients to its patients. But breast milk was the preferred food for many infants, especially those born prematurely. A nurse from the hospital collected four quarts of human breast milk every day from a selected group of women and delivered it to the hospital. [3]

"A pair of substantial mammary glands has the advantage over the two hemispheres of the most learned professor's brain in compounding a nutritious fluid for infants," wrote Dr. Oliver Wendell Holmes in 1867. [4] In the early twentieth century it was thought that children should not have solid food until they were nearly two years old, so they were dependent on milk. However, because their mothers often became pregnant again, most babies had to be weaned long before that age. Cow's milk was the logical substitute for mother's milk.

By 1921 Dr. Charles E. North could report that: "The principles of effective milk control have now been settled to the satisfaction of the scientific world. These principles are sufficiently well understood to form the basis of effective milk legislation and milk regulation. It only remains to educate the people of our cities and towns to a complete realization of the food value of milk (no other food is so vital to the welfare and health of the human race as milk) and of the correct principles of milk control, to bring about a satisfactory solution of the milk problem in every community. Such a result can confidently be expected within the very near future." [5]

New scientific advances made it possible for the Floating's food lab to furnish a formula carefully calibrated to suit the needs of each individual infant. Every patient was examined for the "bacteriology of his or her digestive tract and many cases of intestinal infection without symptoms were greatly benefited by early diagnosis and treatment," Dr. Robert B. Hunt, resident physician, reported in 1913.

Patients who were sent home were given enough milk to ensure that they would have the benefit of twenty-four hours of pure milk—beginning the day they arrived on board. A total of 1,320 quarts of milk, modified for the patients' needs, were sent home that year. The H.P. Hood Dairy supplied this formula to patients and charged only what a family could afford to pay.

DENNY AND BOSWORTH

Bedside and food laboratory records collected on the Floating Hospital over the years constituted the "largest masses of data in existence on infant feeding and the medical results ... our success in the collection and use of breast milk (is) a marked advance in the treatment of the digestive tract in children."[6] The scientific data were contained in a report by members of the visiting staff delivered to a meeting of the New York Academy of Medicine.

Bottling mothers' milk in the food laboratory. Taken in 1906.

The Floating's Dr. Francis Parkman Denny was convinced that adding breast milk, even in small quantities, to the formula of sick infants was

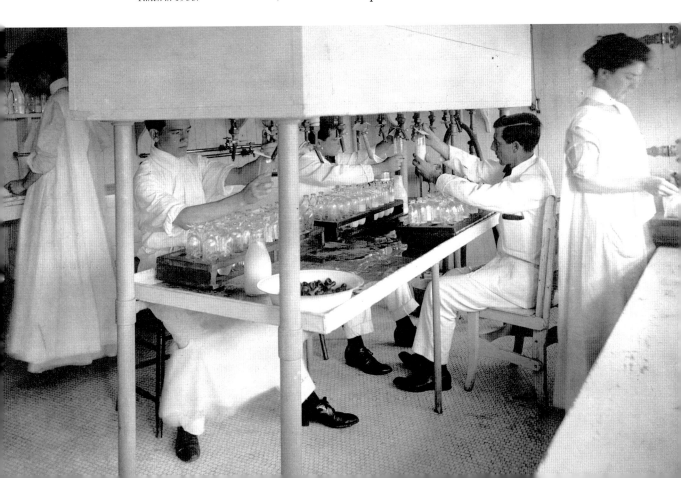

important because of its antibacterial power. Dr. Denny was the driving force behind the continued collection of breast milk from women in the city's poor sections. The women who sold their milk to the hospital were examined to make sure they were in good health.

Dr. Denny knew what to feed the infants, but the man who eventually revolutionized the way babies were fed was Dr. Alfred W. Bosworth,[7] a chemist at the Agricultural Experiment Station in Geneva, New York. Dr. Bosworth first suspected that milk caused intestinal problems while he was studying the chemical processes involved in the ripening of cheese and the make-up of milk. He was living in a house with two young children who were constantly having intestinal problems. He noticed that the children got sick only when they were fed modified cow's milk. When they were nursed, their difficulties ceased. Dr. Bosworth hypothesized that cow's milk, designed for feeding calves, contained too much calcium for children to absorb.

In order to get enough scientific training to solve this problem, Dr. Bosworth came to Harvard Medical School to study physiology, bacteriology, and organic chemistry. In 1912, he was invited by Dr. Otto Folin, a biochemist who studied the patterns of proteins in the blood, to join an investigation of the elements in milk. Their goal was to develop a formula that would eliminate the less-desirable components so that most infants could digest it. After receiving his degree in February 1913, he continued to work with Dr. Folin. Dr. Bosworth returned to Geneva for three years, but then came to the Floating Hospital to assume the position of director of research.

Working in a rented laboratory in the Back Bay, Dr. Bosworth mixed hundreds of formulas, testing the merits of various vegetable oils, concentrations and modifications of protein, and ratios of salts and concentrations of lactose. Metabolic studies were used to evaluate the results of the mixtures.

Dr. Bosworth broke down the components of the milk—separating the cream, evaporating its water content, and adding an acid to the skim milk to isolate the casein, an important nutritional component of milk. He added lime and milk sugar after the milk was strained to preserve the whey. Olive oil was added for extra fat.

The whole mixture was then put into a machine Dr. Bosworth named "The Iron Cow" that broke up the fats by applying three thousand pounds of pressure, which he let escape through a set of valves. Preparing milk this way cost fifteen cents per quart as compared with the thirty-two dollars a quart that was the going rate for breast milk. The milk was mixed twice to ensure that the fat was completely broken up in the mixture to make it more digestible. Dr. Bosworth's analysis showed that he had produced a formula that closely resembled mother's milk.

But he had been unsuccessful in removing excess calcium from his milk mixture. One day, he left a beaker of milk from which he was trying to draw off the calcium on his desk when he was called away. When he returned the next day, the reaction had occurred naturally. He learned that he simply needed to wait for the process to take place.

On the day he was certain that he had come up with the right formula, Dr. Bosworth tested it on some of the sick babies on the Floating under the supervision of Dr. Henry Ingersoll Bowditch, chair of the visiting staff. The next morning, the babies seemed improved. But Dr. Bosworth suspected that he needed to further refine the formula.

The success of Dr. Bosworth's investigations and the increasing attention paid to his research resulted in a substantial donation from "two persons" for equipment and a group of well-appointed laboratories for chemical, biological, and bacteriological investigation. The clinics were established at 38-42 Wigglesworth Street near the Harvard Medical School, as a section of the newly opened Floating's on-shore clinics. Dr. Bosworth worked with Dr. Arthur Kendall and three unnamed chemists. He developed a powdered milk product, which "segregated the constituent elements of milk and reorganized them in proportions practically identical to breast milk."[8]

As Dr. Bowditch bragged in the 1919 annual report: "Our laboratories have so far solved the milk problems which have been under study for some years as to put us in possession of the best substitute for breast milk so all-important in infant feeding."[9]

But by 1921 the trustees no longer "felt justified to stretch the hospital's resources in support of Bosworth's work" and began to seek a way to give the milk formula "to the world without charge." The patents were relinquished in 1922 and the process made available to "all who wish to use them."[10]

Dr. Bosworth left in 1921 to take a job with the Kellogg Company of Battle Creek, Michigan, as chief chemist and director of research, turning his attention to studying the cereal products of the firm. In 1924, a new position with the company that made the popular drink Postum took him to Columbus, Ohio. There, Dr. Bosworth met Stanley Ross of the Moores and Ross Milk and Ice Cream Company. Ross had heard of Dr. Bosworth's infant formula, and the two entered into an agreement with Ross to produce and market the formula.[11]

Moores and Ross invested three hundred thousand dollars to develop the equipment to produce the formula powder. This included an enormous "homogenizer" that was able to mix Dr. Bosworth's formula in large batches. The new powdered milk product was first named Franklin Infant Food because it was manufactured in a converted brewery on Franklin Street in Columbus. Later, the formula's name was changed to SIMILAC because it so closely resembled milk. Dr. Morris Fishbein, the president of the American Medical Association, and the firm's sales manager suggested the name. [12]

An early label listed the ingredients: "Made from fresh skim milk (casein modified) with added lactose, salts, milk fat and vegetable and cod liver oil. Approximate analysis: fats, 27.1%; carbohydrates, 54.4%; protein, 12.3%; ash 3.2%; moisture, 3%; one ounce equals 153.2 calories."

However, not all babies were able to digest even the most carefully manufactured formula. Luckily for those babies, the Floating's lab had worked out another possible solution. In 1922, the Floating labs had perfected a milk-drying machine, which made it possible to dehydrate human milk. This was important during the summer season when there was not always enough fresh breast milk available. The dried milk could be kept on hand and reconstituted when needed for especially sensitive babies. [13]

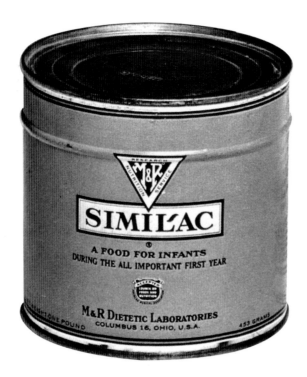

A NOTE ON MILK

PASTEURIZATION

Milk, the "perfect food" for babies and young children, was, at the same time, the perfect medium for the many disease-causing bacteria that resulted in the high mortality rate among infants. Even though by the time the Floating was launched it was understood that milk carried many diseases, pasteurization was not universally adopted for many years.[1]

A French scientist, Blondeau, had observed bacteria in sour milk through his microscope in 1847,[2] but it took Louis Pasteur to connect the organisms with the souring process. In the 1860s, Pasteur demonstrated that abnormal fermentation of wine and beer could be prevented by heating the beverages to about 50° C (122° F) for a few minutes.[3]

Approximately twenty years later, Franz von Soxhelt tried boiling cows' milk to kill bacteria, but the prevention of disease was not the primary purpose for this procedure. It was done to make it possible to transport the milk further and keep it fresh for longer periods of time. In 1886, however, Soxhelt recommended that all cows' milk fed to infants be boiled for thirty-five to forty minutes.[4] "During the process of milking," he said, "particles of manure and other forms of dirt get into the milk and during transportation and handling fermentation (souring) sets in, so that much of our milk is really unfit for consumption before it gets into the stomachs of infants and children." Soxhelt had observed that calves that fed on milk from a trough often suffered from diarrhea.

The first milk law, passed in Massachusetts in 1856, prohibited the adulteration of milk. It had been discovered that cows were being fed slops left over after the making of beer. This so-called swill milk was considered nearly unfit to drink. In 1859, the City of Boston authorized the collection of milk samples for examination and appointed its first milk inspector to enforce regulation against the use of distillery slops. In 1864, Boston prohibited the use of milk from diseased cows.[5]

But the notion that invisible organisms caused diseases that could be spread through milk was not an accepted concept until the 1880s. Robert Koch's invention of solid culture medium in 1881 made it possible to isolate and study bacteria. When Ernest Hart compiled a list[6] of epidemics whose causes could be traced to contaminated milk, the link between milk and disease was firmly established. In 1888, Dr. Augustus Caillé, after a visit to Germany, brought word of Soxhelt's methods of killing these organisms to the United States. Soon, other doctors came to the conclusion that all milk used for feeding infants should be heated to destroy the organisms.

Between 1892 and 1900, there was a scientific breakthrough. Theobald Smith isolated and identified the germs of bovine tuberculosis and determined the temperature at which they were destroyed. Some commercial dairies began to pasteurize milk, but the procedure was not universally adopted. It would be almost ten years (1908) before Chicago became the world's first city to require pasteurization of milk.[7]

In 1892, Dr. Henry L. Coit of Newark, New Jersey, inaugurated a movement to certify milk, and New Jersey became the first state to establish a medical milk commission. Dr. Coit characterized certified milk by "the absence of large numbers of bacteria and the absence of pathogenic varieties; by resistance to fermentation and by its keeping qualities; by constant nutritive values and chemical composition."[8]

After New York established a commission in 1901, other cities followed. By 1906, twenty-seven medical milk commissions had been established in major American cities. In 1907, a National Association of Medical Milk Commissions was organized in Atlantic City, and national standards for certified milk were established.[9] A number of states passed legislation prohibiting the use of the term "certified" except for milk conforming to the national standards and produced under the supervision of authorized medical milk commissions.

It has never been easy to institute a new way of doing things, so it was to be expected that there would be a great deal of resistance to heating milk. Several researchers concluded that, while it was true that there were bacteria in milk, there was not enough evidence that the milk from healthy cows needed to be pasteurized at the dairy. The contamination, these experts declared, had occurred sometime during the transportation of the milk. There was general acceptance of home pasteurization, but the widespread public opposition to commercial pasteurization drove milk producers to secretly pasteurize their product.

Some members of the medical profession were opposed to pasteurization on the grounds that the process lowered the nutritional value of milk, and in 1898 the American Pediatric Society reported cases of scurvy resulting from prolonged feeding with pasteurized milk. The medical community was divided, but a majority of doctors realized that milk infections were dangerous to small children and the pasteurization in the home would never be adequate to protect babies from disease.

In 1906, Dr. Milton J. Rosenau (1869-1946), then director of the United States Marine Hospital Service (MHS) Hygienic Laboratory in Washington, D.C., determined the thermal death point of pathogenic bacteria and established the temperature necessary for the pasteurization of milk. Dr. Charles. E. North, a leader in gaining public acceptance of pasteurization, established a new way of pasteurizing milk called the "holding method." It was being tested in the largest pasteurizing plant in New York City using a newly designed machine. The holding method was soon in wide use for pasteurizing milk and, in a short time, replaced the earlier flash method. Later Dr. North was instrumental in the passage of laws making milk pasteurization mandatory around the country.

FEEDING STATIONS

In 1893, Nathan Straus, a New York philanthropist and co-owner of R. H. Macy & Company department store, opened feeding stations in that city to provide pasteurized milk and formula to the poor. Straus sold both eight-ounce bottles of milk and six-ounce bottles of a formula consisting of 2 percent fat, 2 percent protein, and 7 percent sugar. Later, the formula was modified as ¼ ounce of table salt and ten ounces of white cane sugar were added to each gallon of milk and gallon of barley water.[10] The Straus feeding stations, which operated at his expense for twenty-six years, featured a milk bottle cleverly designed to prevent contamination of its contents. The necks and shoulders of the bottles sloped for easy washing, and because of their spheroid bottoms, the bottles could not be stored upright or without a stopper.[11] In the summer months from 1890 to 1892, 13,201 children under five had died in New York City. Almost half of them succumbed to cholera infantum. The Straus depots greatly reduced this mortality rate.[12]

Straus benefited from the advice of Dr. North, who played a major role in setting standards for the stations. Drs. Rowland G. Freeman and Abraham Jacobi were also early advocates of pasteurization. Always a champion of new ideas, Dr. Jacobi praised Soxhelt's methods of pasteurization in a paper read before the Public Health Association of New York.

Some feeding stations only provided milk prepared according to formulas and pasteurized it in the nursing bottles. The bottles were distributed with instructions to the mothers on the importance of keeping milk cool and clean. Other milk dispensaries distributed pasteurized milk in quart bottles and sent nurses into the homes to teach the mothers how to prepare formula and take care of the baby at home.[13]

The Walker-Gordon Farm[14] in Needham, Massachusetts, and its first laboratory, established in Boston in 1891, produced and used its clean, modified milk to prepare the formula developed by Dr. Thomas Morgan Rotch[15] (¼ part cream; ½ part milk; one part water; one measure {³/₃₈ dram} lactose; and ¹/₁₆ part lime water per eight-ounce mixture). Other Walker-Gordon labs were eventually established around the country to provide sterilized, pure milk products.

When the New York Milk Committee was organized in 1907 by The Association for Improving the Condition of the Poor, the average infant mortality for the previous ten years in New York City had been 153 per 1,000. The committee's objectives were the reduction of infant death and improvement of the New York City milk supply. It became the model for similar groups all over the country.[16]

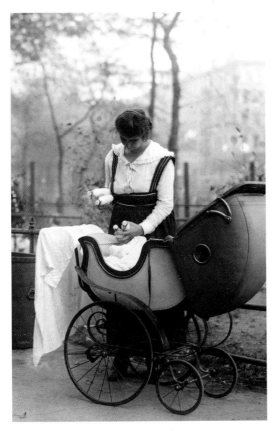

A mother taking milk home. Taken circa 1900.

By 1911, the New York Milk Committee had opened thirty-one milk depots in various New York City locations to demonstrate that, by dispensing pasteurized milk to thousands of infants and educating their mothers about the importance of pasteurization, there was a measureable reduction in infant mortality. In 1912, the City of New York took over their operation. Soon, milk stations on the New York model had been established in many parts of the country.[17]

In 1910, the Boston Milk and Baby Hygiene Association set up the Sun Court Street Stations near the Floating pier. These stations were open at 4:30 in the afternoon so that mothers leaving the Floating with their babies could obtain milk for the night.[18]

But it was still necessary to encourage the milk industry to institute reliable pasteurization methods. In 1908, the New York Milk Committee, at the recommendation of Dr. North, set up a large experimental milk station in rural Homer, New York, to show dairy farmers how they could economically produce commercially pasteurized milk. The practice gradually spread to all the large cities of the country.[19]

Bacterial standards for safe milk were established when the American Public Health Association published its guidelines for the bacterial testing of milk, and that laid the foundation for the establishment of municipal and commercial milk laboratories.[20]

During the first decade of the twentieth century, the campaign for pasteurized milk picked up speed quickly. Advocates of raw milk began to be overwhelmed by the evidence of the effectiveness of pasteurization. From 1907 to 1910, there was a decided drop in epidemics of typhoid fever, scarlet fever, and diphtheria, as well as a drop in infant mortality wherever pasteurization was established.

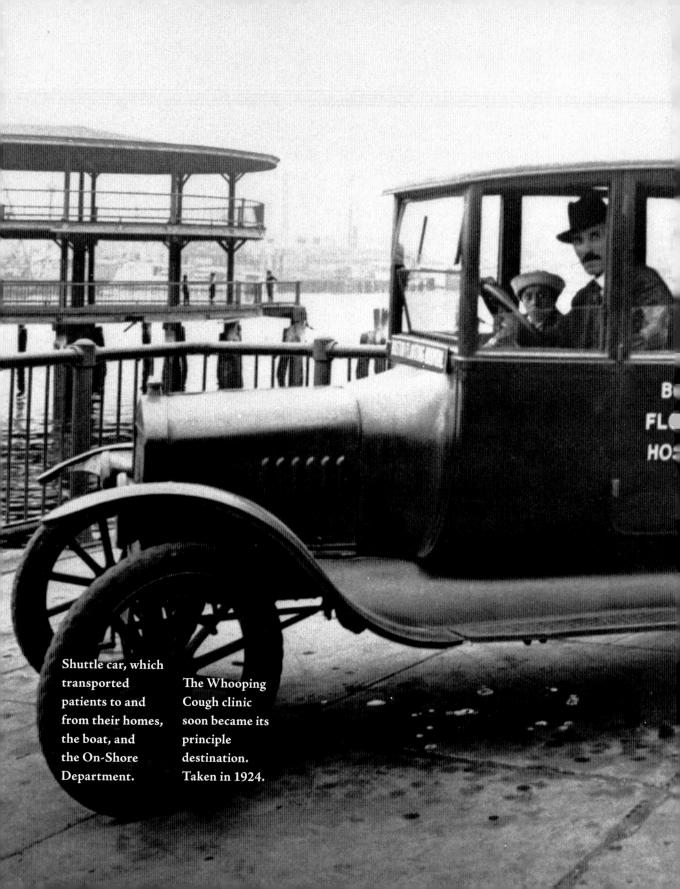

Shuttle car, which transported patients to and from their homes, the boat, and the On-Shore Department.

The Whooping Cough clinic soon became its principle destination. Taken in 1924.

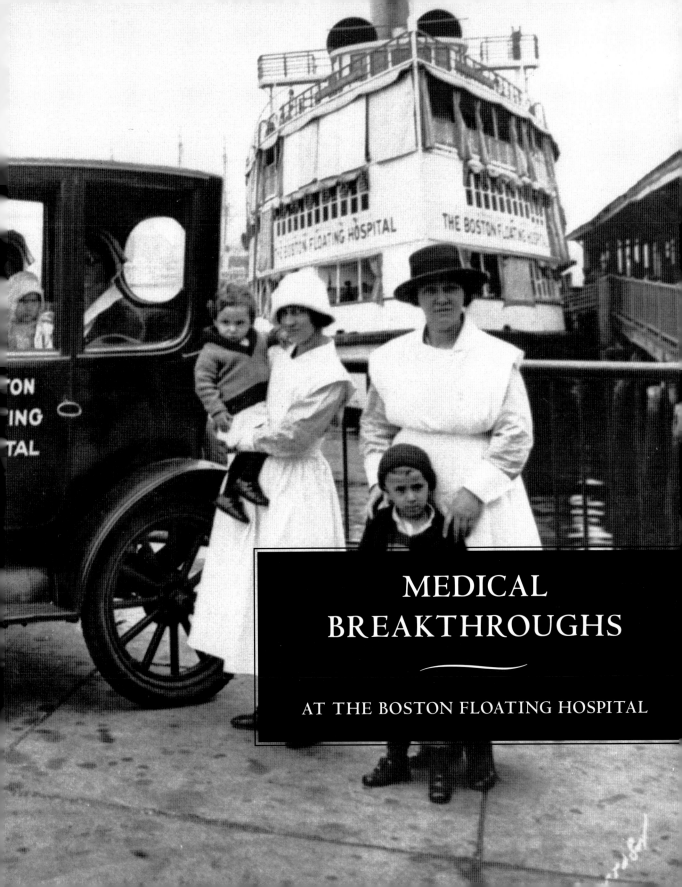

MEDICAL BREAKTHROUGHS

AT THE BOSTON FLOATING HOSPITAL

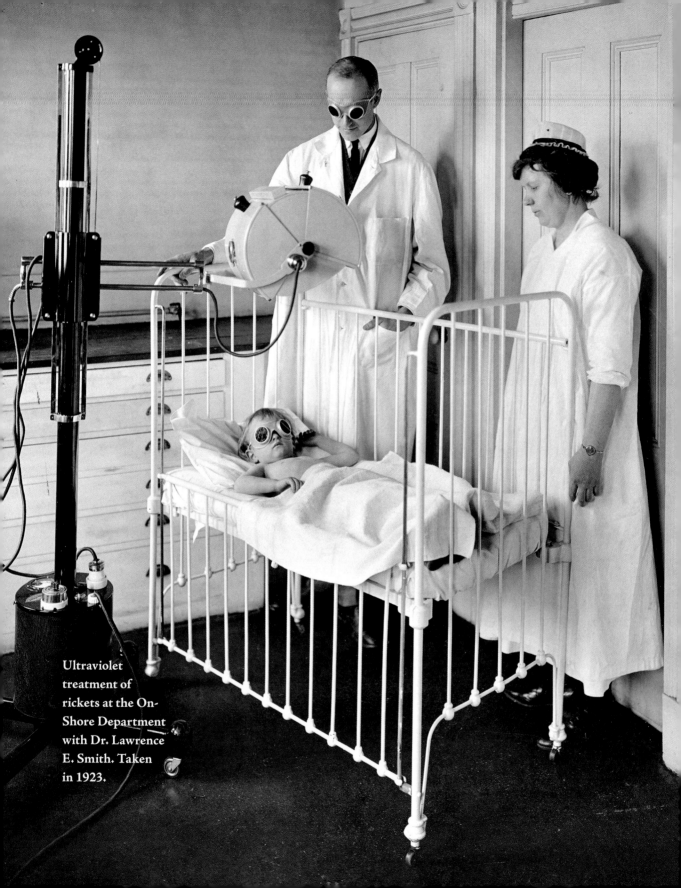

Ultraviolet treatment of rickets at the On-Shore Department with Dr. Lawrence E. Smith. Taken in 1923.

MEDICAL BREAKTHROUGHS
AT THE BOSTON FLOATING HOSPITAL

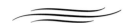

While medical research was not the main objective of the Floating, it presented its doctors and nurses with a unique set of patients. It was uncommon to see so many children with similar diseases in one place at one time. Having their collective symptoms and treatment results at their finger-tips, doctors were able to make advances in the diagnoses and treatment of not only cholera infantum, but also many other childhood diseases. The work done at the Floating directly resulted in the expansion of the field of pediatrics, major advances in pediatric nutrition, and the invention of infant formula.

While many major advancements took place on the new boat, it was the work aboard the *Clifford* that paved the way. The food lab and the Floating's sterilization techniques were ahead of their time.

Evolution of the Food Lab

The modified milk department, established in 1896, became the food laboratory in 1902. Charles E. Buck, a graduate pharmacist, and Dr. Hibbert H. Hill of the Boston Board of Health demonstrated how to test the purity of all the foods given to the babies. During the Floating's 1902 season "nearly ideal results were obtained."

Fresh milk and cream, produced in sanitary conditions and kept cold, had been successfully shipped to the Paris Exposition in 1900 from dairy farms in the United States. The next year, the Deerfoot Farm Company in Southborough, Massachusetts, had begun to ship milk to the Floating. This milk was poured into special containers immediately after milking and was received at the Floating three or four hours later. After being analyzed for bacteria by Dr. Hill, it was used without further sterilization.[1]

Placing the various elements of the formula in separate receptacles and filling each feeding bottle with the proper proportions of food solved the problem of feeding so many babies at one time. The food left the laboratory at a high temperature, but the time it took to get to the child was carefully monitored so that it was at the proper warmth when it was received. This feeding marathon occurred simultaneously at six different points on the boat every two hours.

In 1902, the Floating received contamination-free milk directly from Walker-Gordon Farm in Needham, Massachusetts.[2] The control of flies, sterilization of the hospital's laundry by formalin, and the cleansing of the hands of doctors and nurses were now completely routine on the Floating. Further, the hospital's laboratory examined the blood and urine of every patient to rule out infectious diseases. A newly inaugurated system of record keeping contributed to the overall modernization of the hospital's functions.

Increasingly, the most important area of the hospital's work was the food department. It made daily tests of the purity of milk, cream, sugar, water, sugar solution, and of all the various foods prepared. The milk from Walker-Gordon cows continued to be remarkably free of germs upon examination by the food lab. To further modernize the food preparation, the atmospheric plant now furnished refrigeration for the food laboratory. (This worked well when the weather was relatively cool, but when it wasn't, the demands on the system prevented it from performing this additional duty.)

Sterilization and Pathology

Infection was always the greatest fear of the doctors working in the confined quarters of the *Clifford*. From the very first trip on, referring doctors had been instructed not to send any child with an infectious disease to the boat, and the staff worked diligently to prevent infection on board. In 1901, a campaign against flies, recently recognized as disease bearers, was added to these efforts.

John Collins Warner, who had seen the results of Joseph Lister's carbolic spray and chemical cleansing of the operational field in Glasgow, Scotland, had introduced antisepsis to Boston in 1869. (Lister went on to develop a sanitizing product that is popular to this day and bears his name: Listerine.) It was not in common use, however, until the end of the decade. Boston City Hospital's first antiseptic operation was performed in 1879. By the late 1880s, asepsis was replacing antisepsis. In 1891, the Boston Children's Hospital refitted its operating room with aseptic furnishing and an up-to-date sterilization system, which required a scrupulously clean surgical environment rather than relying on a disinfectant spray during operations. Antisepsis and asepsis combated germ concentrations and made hospital surgery relatively safe.[3] The Floating was scrupulous about keeping the premises as antiseptic as possible.

In order to keep the ever-changing linens free of contamination, even before they were sent to the laundry, they were all sterilized in large steam cylinders controlled by the health board. The entire staff washed their hands and took other special precautions before coming in contact with patients. Largely due to these efforts, during the 1901 summer season not a single case of infection was contracted on board the Floating. This "has thrown some light upon the question of what the much talked about 'hospitalism' in infants' hospitals is all about," said the 1901 annual report, referring to the widespread fear of infection that caused most people to be terrified of being admitted to a hospital. As sterilization began to be introduced universally at the end of the century, this fear began to decline.

In 1901, the Floating added a pathology laboratory to help make diagnoses. The lab had been squeezed into a space created by closing one entrance of Ward B and blocking off one half of the main stairway. While it was just big enough to permit two men to use their microscopes at one time, the pathology work was increasingly important to the hospital. It would become a more central part of the Floating's work in the future, but even in the early days it functioned to the hospital's benefit. During the 1901 season, the lab was able to discover a case of diphtheria in one young patient, a baby who was immediately transferred to the City Hospital to avoid infecting any of the other children.

With the pathology lab results in hand, doctors could now differentiate between intestinal diseases as well; they no longer had to lump all these infections under "cholera infantum." The list of the 1901 season's intestinal illnesses shows a greater sophistication in diagnosis.[4]

Air Conditioning and Air Quality

Even on the water, the weather could be oppressive, especially to those small children who were suffering from intestinal diseases. The innovators who put a hospital on a barge, however, did not accept this as an insurmountable problem.

In 1898, the directors began to look for a way to "modify the air in our wards in such a way that our patients shall have dry air of moderate temperature which shall be uniform irrespective of the weather." They heard that Lowney & Co., chocolate manufacturers in Mansfield, Massachusetts, had "modified" the air in their factory at a cost of $20,000.[5] If twenty thousand dollars could be spent to cool chocolates, the Floating should not hesitate to find a way to reduce the temperature in its wards in order to save the lives of children, the directors stated. All estimates showed the Floating could do this for far less than Lowneys had spent. Contributions earmarked for this purpose were immediately solicited. "As yet no precedent for this exists. But it is difficult to see how such a result can be otherwise than beneficial and should be so in a high degree. The expense is moderate, about $5,000. The matter is under advisement at present and the medical staff most sincerely hopes that the plan may be realized," they reported to their potential contributors.[6]

It would be an extraordinary addition to the hospital, to any hospital, at that time, but the dedicated board of trustees had decided it was a necessity and consulted an engineer from the Massachusetts Institute of Technology. By the following year, the new "Atmospheric Plant" had been installed. The 1899 annual report described it as such: "The object of this plant is, taking the air in its varying conditions of temperature and percentage of moisture, to reduce its relative humidity to about fifty percent and to raise or lower its temperature to a desirable point, which is, in a hospital ward, about 74° F." The results showing the success of the plant can never be enumerated, as there is no doubt that a great many patients owed their lives to the cool and dry air furnished to them when the natural air condition was unbearable.[7]

The Floating's 1900 History and Report observed, "The air is first received into a large ventilating pipe projecting about seven feet above the upper deck, and by means of a revolving fan is carried over a series of pipes in which brine, at a temperature of about 10° Fahrenheit is circulating. The brine in these pipes is kept constantly cool by means of an ice machine of eight tons capacity, a special pump being used to circulate the brine. Contact with these cold pipes reduces the temperature of the air considerably below the point desired for the wards, and in so doing precipitates the moisture or, in other words, dries the air. The air is then passed over pipes heated by steam and thus raised to the proper temperature for distribution to the wards. The pipes for the wards are large, so that the current of air is not a violent one and the outlets are so arranged that no draughts of air can affect the patients. The wards, of course, are tightly closed."[8]

So it was that in 1899 a small hospital, established only five years earlier and functioning on a remodeled barge in Boston Harbor, became the first hospital in America to air condition its wards.

During the next two years, the Floating adjusted the air conditioning system and conducted studies to assess the importance of air conditioning on the patients. Because it was believed that a combination of natural and conditioned air was best, the window openings on the boat were as large as possible. In cooler weather, only natural air was used, while during hotter days, a combination of natural and conditioned air was employed. It seems obvious now that this combination must have cut down the efficiency and put a strain on the system.

Simon Flexner

Simon Flexner was one of the most important American scientists of the early twentieth century. His research in poliomyelitis led to the identification of the virus that caused the disease, the discovery of the method by which it is transmitted from person to person, and the method by which it enters the body. He also developed a serum for cerebrospinal meningitis. In the summer of 1903, Flexner was the director of laboratories of the recently established Rockefeller Institute for Medical Research in Manhattan. He subsequently served as the director of the Rockefeller Institute from 1920 to 1935.[9]

In 1903, he chose the Floating to be a proving ground for a serum that held the promise of curing dysentery. On a mission to the Philippines in 1899, Flexner had isolated the bacillus that is the cause of tropical dysentery. The germ now bears his name: *Shigella flexneri.* The serum he developed had been used in adult dysentery during several epidemics in Japan.[10] It had proved absolutely harmless in adults, but Flexner still needed to test it on children. In those days, parental consent was not needed for such trials, and Flexner's reputation was such that the hospital's staff eagerly accepted his offer.

Under Flexner's supervision the serum was tested only on those patients with severe diarrhea in whom the dysentery bacillus was found. Dr. Arthur Kendall, a bacteriologist, was the chief investigator, and Dr. Paul A. Lewis was his assistant. Dr. Kendall furnished the Rockefeller Institute reports of thirty-five cases. Unfortunately, the serum injections were "almost entirely negative in their results," but while they didn't work, the experience did confirm that the serum had no ill effect. There was hope that a stronger serum would be available the following summer.

CHOLERA INFANTUM

For many years, cholera infantum remained the major cause for admission to the Floating. In 1893, the number of childhood deaths from that disease in Massachusetts was 2,704, or 11.1 per 10,000 living population. Of these cases, 88.6 percent occurred in the months of July, August, and September.[11] The disease was so named because the violence of its symptoms resembled those of cholera. (It was also called "Cholera Morbus," especially when the patient was an adult; Theodore Roosevelt was once diagnosed with the disease).

The History of Cholera Infantum

Dr. Benjamin Rush, (1746-1813), in a paper delivered in 1777, described cholera infantum's symptoms as frequent, explosive, watery, and sometimes bloody stools, accompanied by vomiting resulting in rapid and great emaciation.[12] Considered one of the ablest physicians of his time, Dr. Rush, a close friend of Benjamin Franklin, was one of five doctors who signed the Declaration of Independence.

By the mid-nineteenth century, the medical profession suspected that milk was the culprit in this often-fatal disease, but until the milk supply could be protected from bacteria, there was little people could do to prevent the disease. Doctors had developed various methods for treating children who were afflicted, but most of these methods failed.

In 1825, Dr. William Potts Dewees (1768-1841) said that children infected with cholera infantum should be sent to the country. Those who couldn't go should have their stomachs "tranquilized," meaning: "The irritating contents of the stomach should be removed by encouraging the infant to puke by draughts of warm, or even cold, water, where the warm will not be drunk, until no foreign substance appears in the matter thrown up." Then patients should get "a teaspoon full of strong coffee, without sugar or milk, every fifteen minutes." If that didn't work, he recommended calomel. If symptoms persisted, laudanum was added to calomel, followed by bleeding or the application of leeches over the stomach.[13]

In his *Treatise on Children*, published in 1833, Dr. John Eberle (1788–1838) described "atmospheric heat, dentition (teething), and the impure air of cities," as the cause of cholera infantum.[14] He applied leeches to the temples or induced small blisters either behind the ears or on the back of the neck, and he advised that small doses of calomel and ipecac, as well as "stimulating poultices," be placed over the abdomen. He noted that children with the disease often exhibited a craving for salty food. This was probably due to the dehydration induced by the disease.

In a 1939 article about the history of pediatrics,[15] Grover F. Powers (1887-1960) wrote, "The summer complaint was the principal disease (in the nineteenth century) and the principal weapons against it were tea, barley water, protein milk, floating hospitals, and seaside or country sanitaria."

In his textbook on childhood diseases,[16] Dr. George F. Still (1868-1941) described the treatment of cholera infantum. He was critical of the physician who, he wrote, in many cases of acute summer diarrhea "sees the infant perhaps in the morning, gives his orders and says that he'll return the next

Metabolism crib with the coverings drawn aside and crib details. Taken in 1917.

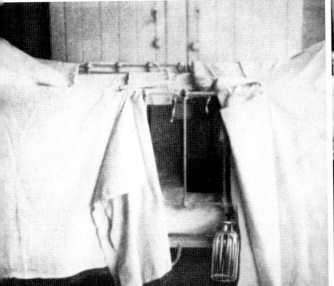
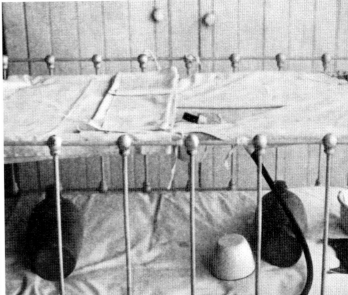

day." The "infant passes rapidly from bad to worse; if the food or drug which is doing no good is continued for several hours, the chance of saving the infant's life is lost. It may be necessary for the doctor to see the infant twice or even thrice in a day to adopt his measure to the changing and pressing needs of the infant."

"In the acute stage," Dr. Still advised, "the prohibition of all milk ... substituting at once some much weaker form of nutriment which may relieve bowel from irritating residue." He suggested "albumen-water, barley-water (or, better, rice-water), weak veal or chicken broth, ordinary tea freshly infused and made very weak ... the urgent need is fluid."

Dr. Still was adamant that "no looseness of the bowels in an infant, however slight it may appear, is to be regarded lightly" in the summer months.

Cholera Infantum on *The Boston Floating Hospital*

The Floating took great pains to care for the children with cholera infantum. Below is a description of how nurses and doctors on the Floating cared for children with this ailment from the magazine *The Nurse* in an article entitled, "A Day on the White Ship of Mercy." [17]

"Upon the admission of such a case (infectious diarrhea) a bacteriological examination is made in the vessel's laboratory to determine whether the cause is the Flexner or the gas bacillus. These children are put on sterile water, and if a preliminary smear examination of the stool points toward gas bacilli the patient is at once put on buttermilk and water; but, on the other hand, if Flexner bacilli are indicated as the cause of the trouble, the food is made up of barley water and lactose. The final diagnosis cannot be made earlier than three days, but whether the case is one of Flexner or gas bacillus dysentery, the child is put at this time on buttermilk and water, equal parts, with the addition, in the first class, of barley water to seventy-five per cent and lactose to six per cent.

"Babies suffering from chronic intestinal indigestion, babies on whom all sorts of foods have been tried at home without success, and premature infants are fed with breast milk, generally diluted with water or with whey. Many babies in collapse from acute intestinal indigestion, the so-called intestinal intoxication cases, do very well on dilutions of breast milk and whey in very small quantities at very frequent intervals for the first three or four days."

MEDICAL ADVANCES AND RESEARCH

The abundance of patients provided doctors and nurses on the Floating with ample chances to test new theories and methods. These opportunities led to advances in both medicine and the manner in which children were treated.

One of the research projects mentioned in the same article in *The Nurse*[18] was a study of the metabolism of infants who had been cured of intestinal infections. A special bed had been constructed for the study, and although it sounds like a torture chamber, readers are assured that "a more contented group of babies could not be imagined than those who were the subjects of this investigation." Three photos accompanying the article show the specially constructed crib, the equipment that collected the specimens used in the study, and a baby who seems at least placid, if not contented.

The baby rested on a cloth sling suspended over the top of the crib. The child was held in a fixed position by a bellyband, and his or her legs, encased in long stockings, were pinned to the sling. Coverings draped the crib, and hot water jugs placed beneath the child kept it warm. For seven days—if we can believe the author—the baby stayed in this crib in that position while a bowl suspended under an opening in the center of the sling captured his or her "dejections." Urine was collected through a tube and fed into a container suspended on the side of the crib. The child was checked often for chafing, and absolute cleanliness was maintained.

A contented subject of metabolic research. Taken in 1917.

The urine and feces of the infants in the study underwent quantitative, chemical, and bacteriological analyses, and careful records of what the child ingested were also kept. The study hoped to discover the causes of gastroenteritis and to devise more effective treatment for this disease.

The article also describes the incubator for premature infants used on the Floating. The author praises the hospital for participating in the new trend that turned away from enclosed and artificially ventilated incubators. The incubator was simply a crib enclosed with sheets. There was an opening in the sheets above the infant's head. The baby, dressed

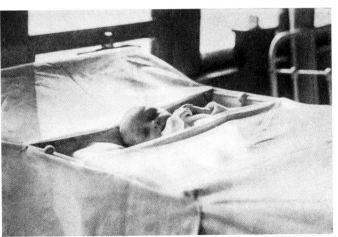

in an "incubator jacket" resembling a quilted bag with a hood, was kept inside the crib that was heated by hot water jugs. The temperature inside the incubator was brought down to the outside temperature as soon as the baby seemed able to survive in normal conditions. Ventilation in the incubator was adjusted simply by enlarging or narrowing the opening in the sheet so that the "sea breeze (could give) an ample change of air." Among the many skills taught to the nurses in the hospital's program of ward instruction was how to make the premature jackets.

In the 1913 annual report, Dr. Arthur Kendall listed the contributions of the hospital during the three years since its scientific work began in earnest: [19]

1910

Shortened bacteriological diagnosis of dysentery by 24 hours

Established Gas Bacillus as predominating organism
in certain dysenteries

Demonstrated an easy clinical test for Gas Bacillus infection

Established a theory for treatment in such cases in the form of buttermilk
and demonstrated its use in such cases

Shortened starvation period for all dysenteries

Established the use of Dextrose Saline solution in the form of infusions for stimulation in cases showing collapse or depletion (dehydration)

1911

Isolated the Shiga Bacillus from the blood (first known case on record)

Established the clinical position of irrigation in cases of dysentery

Tested the use of constant seepage

Demonstrated the prevalence of Pyelitis in Streptococcus infection of the intestinal tract

1912

Demonstrated the use of high proteins in Gas Bacillus infections

Demonstrated the dangerous treatment of administration of lactose
or sugars in such cases

1913

Further demonstrated the use of high proteins in dysenteries not
Flexner, Shiga nor Streptococcus Etiology

Demonstrated the use of maltose as a food to be easily absorbed,
digested and assimilated

Over a period of years, the Floating was recognized as a national research center for the study of intestinal diseases in children. A bacteriological lab had been established in 1910 at Harvard Medical School under the direction of Dr. Otto Folin, America's first clinical biochemist, then a professor of biochemistry. Through the "kindness of a certain friend of the Floating," Dr. Kendall was continuing the work on the bacteriological study of childhood diseases of the digestive tract that he had begun in 1910. Dr. Henry Ingersoll Bowditch, chairman of the visiting staff, was convinced that this research would eventually enable physicians to diagnose cases from a combination of the clinical, bacteriological, and chemical points of view in order to treat patients more scientifically.

By the end of the first two decades of the twentieth century, the number of intestinal disorders of the sort seen by the Floating was steadily decreasing. The pasteurization of the city's milk supply, which was made compulsory in 1921, as well as the improvement of hygiene and sewerage, played important roles in reducing the morbidity among the youngest of the hospital's patients. In 1922, only 64 out of the 221 permanent patients and only 38 day patients had serious intestinal problems. By 1924, only 8 of the 230 permanent patients had intestinal diarrhea.[20]

The Floating began to shift its attention to the study of nutritional diseases, such as rickets, that had supplanted cholera infantum as a leading cause of disease in its patients. By raising the maximum age of day patients to eight years in 1922, doctors could expand their investigation of nutritional diseases to include children who had left infancy and early childhood.

"Many of the children on the Day Deck showed various manifestations of rickets," reported Dr. Robert Hunt, the resident physician, in 1923. "Some were in early stages of the disease, others showed backward (slow) development, while still others were markedly deformed. By means of carefully regulated diets, graded exercises and exposure to the direct sunlight we were able to produce beneficial results."[21]

X-RAYS AND WHOOPING COUGH

While the Floating's staff always had their patients' interests at the forefront of their procedures, not every medical breakthrough was beneficial in the long term. Hindsight and subsequent scientific advances show that one such example was the use of X-rays in the treatment of whooping cough.

The Floating was just a year old when on November 8, 1895, William Conrad Roentgen discovered X-rays while conducting experiments with vacuum tubes. Faith in the therapeutic value of X-rays continued for many years before the full knowledge of the danger from exposure to radiation was known; the miracle of X-ray technology outweighed caution.

Because whooping cough was among the most dangerous of the children's diseases, the hospital began a year-long study of the curative effect of X-rays in the treatment of whooping cough in 1922. An outpatient clinic was opened to pursue this work.[22] The program, which was under the direction of Dr. Bowditch, began when a mother begged him to help her sick child, and it occurred to him that X-rays might be an effective way to treat this infection. A report to the Baby Hygiene Association in 1923 by Dr. Lawrence W. Smith, resident physician, demonstrates how important this investigation was considered by the medical establishment at the time:[23]

"In the spring of 1923, three hundred and fifty cases (of whooping cough) were seen and given an average of three X-ray treatments at two-day intervals. Between seventy-five and eighty percent so treated felt the treatment was of definite benefit. In general it was found that the best results followed in the younger patients and the earlier in the course of the disease that the treatment was started.

"The success of treatment was so definite in this preliminary survey that X-ray men in various parts of the country have taken it up and enthusiastic reports from them suggest that we have been very conservative in our attitude. The co-operation of the health departments of several of the municipalities of Greater Boston has been secured and a similar campaign is being carried out along even broader lines.

"More intensive study is being carried out in the wards of the on-shore department which were opened in the fall of 1923 for this purpose. The object of this work is to make more careful scientific observations under adequately controlled conditions.

"Bacteriological, serological, and pathological, as well as clinical studies are being carried on intensively to demonstrate that, by means of the X-ray, control of one of the most dreaded infections of infancy can be secured.

"The on-shore clinic was reopened in the early autumn and ward patients were admitted for intensive study; and research work for the scientific determination of the results of the treatment will be continued into the coming year."

A high-frequency electromagnetic current machine was installed for the "diathermic treatment" of several diseases such as pneumonia. These machines had been used at the on-shore clinic in conjunction with the whooping cough investigation and were transferred to the boat in the summer. The whooping cough project continued. By 1924, one thousand cases had been treated with X-rays, and since 80 percent of these children showed improvement within

X-ray treatment of whooping cough at the On-Shore Department. Taken circa 1920.

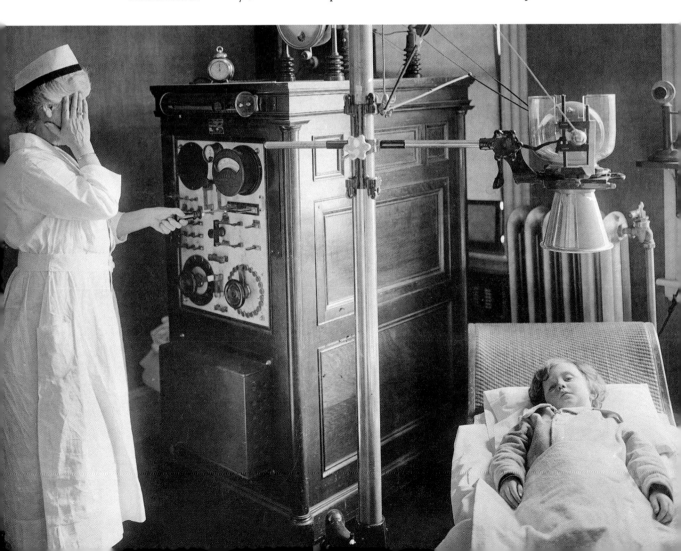

a short time of being exposed to the X-rays, the doctors were coming to the conclusion that this was a good method for treating this disease. Sadly, the danger of exposing children to ionizing radiation was simply not known at that time. Meanwhile, the doctors were also engaged in bacteriological studies, examining the blood of children with whooping cough for changes that might assist them in early diagnosis.

By 1926, the whooping cough clinic had been in operation for four years and had attracted attention nationally and abroad. After attending a conference on whooping cough therapies at the Serum Institute in Copenhagen, Dr. Smith reported that the work at the Floating was more advanced than what he had seen in Denmark.[24]

In 1926, more than fifteen hundred cases of whooping cough were seen at the on-shore clinic. Because the Contagious Diseases Department of the City Hospital was so overcrowded with other infectious illnesses that they had been unable to care for whooping cough cases for the past two years, the Floating had become the only Boston hospital dealing with cases of whooping cough.[25]

Diathermy treatment of pneumonia at the On-Shore Department. Taken in 1923.

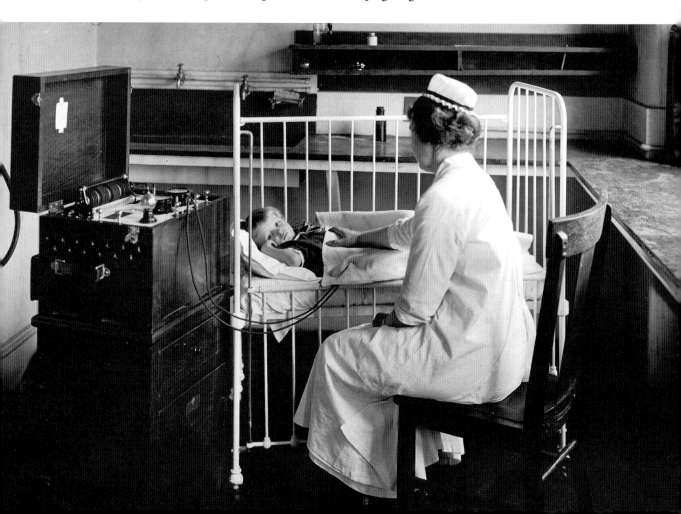

The clinic not only gave X-ray treatments, it also offered a newly developed vaccine to its patients and to children who had been exposed to the disease. The vaccine proved quite effective. Out of 255 children who had been exposed to the disease and were inoculated, 176 did not get whooping cough, and the rest had less serious forms of the disease. Children who suffered from bronchopneumonia, one of the complications of whooping cough, received both X-rays and vaccines. Only 1 percent of the children in this study died of whooping cough, the lowest percentage in any published report. From 1908 to 1925, the death rate from whooping cough was 7.4 percent. In three years, the mortality had dropped 75 percent.[26]

SOLARIUM

The Floating increasingly explored new ways of treating childhood diseases. During the 1920s, Americans became excited about the many new technologies that had become available. The medical profession began to use these new discoveries and inventions to treat patients. The healing powers of the sun were now augmented by the use of a popular ultraviolet apparatus, the so-called sun lamp. The device was used as a supplement to heliotherapy (exposure to the sun) in climates where there was little sun, as well as in the winter. But it was also used in the Floating's on-shore department. The resident physician reported in 1925 that this treatment was no longer in an experimental stage but "accepted generally as being of definite value in arresting the progress of certain nutritional disturbances."[27]

During the summer aboard the boat, the sun had long been considered a primary and natural source of healing. In a new solarium erected on the hurricane deck, children were treated to gradually increasing doses of direct sunlight. A railing five feet high enclosed the after part of the deck, which was lined with canvas to prevent any breeze from blowing directly on the children. (It was generally believed that exposure to the sun was beneficial but direct breezes were dangerous.) At first, the project was under the supervision of Dr. Horace LoGrasso of Perrysburg, New York, a proponent of Rolier's Alpine Sun Method, an improved version of the ultraviolet sun lamp developed in Switzerland in 1916 by a group of physicians. Then Ms. Catherine Wellington, who spent a month at Dr. LoGrasso's hospital learning his techniques, took over.[28]

By the end of the season, reported the resident physician in 1924, patients exposed to the sun in this way were "deeply pigmented from head to toe and brown as berries." Periodically, these children were examined with X-rays and "improvement was noted in their bones" corresponding to the amount of suntan they had developed.[29] The danger of exposing children to that much sunlight was not known at that time.

EXPANDED DEPARTMENTS AND CLINICS

The doctors on the *Clifford* focused primarily on cholera infantum, but as the years went by, the patients' illnesses became more and more diverse. Soon, doctors began to specialize and form more focused departments and clinics on the boat.

In 1916, Dr. Walter C. Miner, the hospital's stomatologist, instituted a new line of study. All patients would now have their primary teeth examined and cared for if need be.[30]

That 1926 season, a nose and throat service was opened on board, and it was now possible for the doctors to remove infected tonsils and adenoids from both day and permanent patients. A dental service was also established. Most of the doctors were convinced that nose and throat infections and dental problems were all implicated in severe intestinal infections.[31]

Special clinics for cardiac cases, those patients with postural and nutritional defects, and those patients who were thought to need heliotherapy because of rickets or other orthopedic defects were all established on board.

The Floating continued to grow as demand for its services increased. In 1935, a new infant ward was set up. Graduate nurses were now able to take a six-month course of study at the Floating. In 1937, a three-month course for students of affiliated nursing schools was offered, and the hospital added a new room for medical records and a library.

"We'd take some mattresses up to the hurricane deck and then we'd bring the babies up with nothing on but a hat on the head, the little white hat to protect their head and a diaper. And we'd expose them to the direct rays of the sun for a measured length of time for the treatment of rickets."
—Harold Freeman. *Early treatment of rickets was a strong dose of sunshine. Later, advances in science led to heliotherapy labs. Taken circa 1920s.*

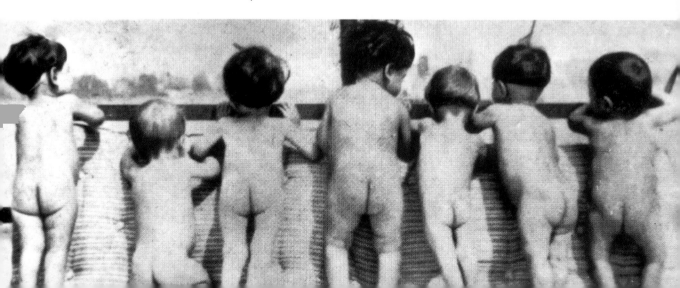

During the 1940s and 1950s, pediatric hospitals had to deal with many illnesses that have essentially been eliminated today, either through immunization or surgical or medical intervention. Once firmly established on shore, the Floating had a special infectious disease section where children of all ages, from newborns to teenagers, were kept in isolation from the other patients. Many suffered from the complications of measles, whooping cough, and other childhood ailments that are rare today. In addition, children died of a form of leukemia that is largely curable today. The field of pediatric cardiology was in its early stages, and the pediatric open-heart operations that are now performed with regularity were considered experimental at the time.

POLIO

In the summers of 1954 and 1955, America experienced the worst polio epidemic in its history. In Massachusetts, there were 3,600 cases statewide and 677 in Boston alone. In the month of July 1954, sixteen people died of the disease in the city.[32] At the height of the epidemic, all the patients were moved out of the Floating into the adult unit of the Center Building on Nassau Street to make room for sixty polio patients. Calls for nurses to help augment the staff at the Floating and at all other hospitals went out over the city. It was an asset that Dr. Louis Weinstein, one of the country's foremost authorities on polio, was chief of infectious diseases at the Floating during this time.

Two of the children of James Collins, a Boston city councilman, were hospitalized in the Floating. Not long after they were admitted, Collins said that he thought he was ill. When he arrived, the diagnosis was clear; he also had polio. His walk into the hospital director's office was the last he ever managed without assistance. Collins was admitted to the adult unit, and after convalescence and rehabilitation, he was able to walk with two canes. He soon ran a successful campaign for mayor in spite of his paralysis.

The 1954-1955 polio epidemic may have been the worst in Boston's history, but it was also the last. In 1955, Jonas Salk developed his vaccine, and polio ceased to

Junior League volunteers assist in hydrotherapy treatment to a young polio patient in the new, five-thousand-dollar Hubbard tank, purchased by Junior League contributions. Date unknown.

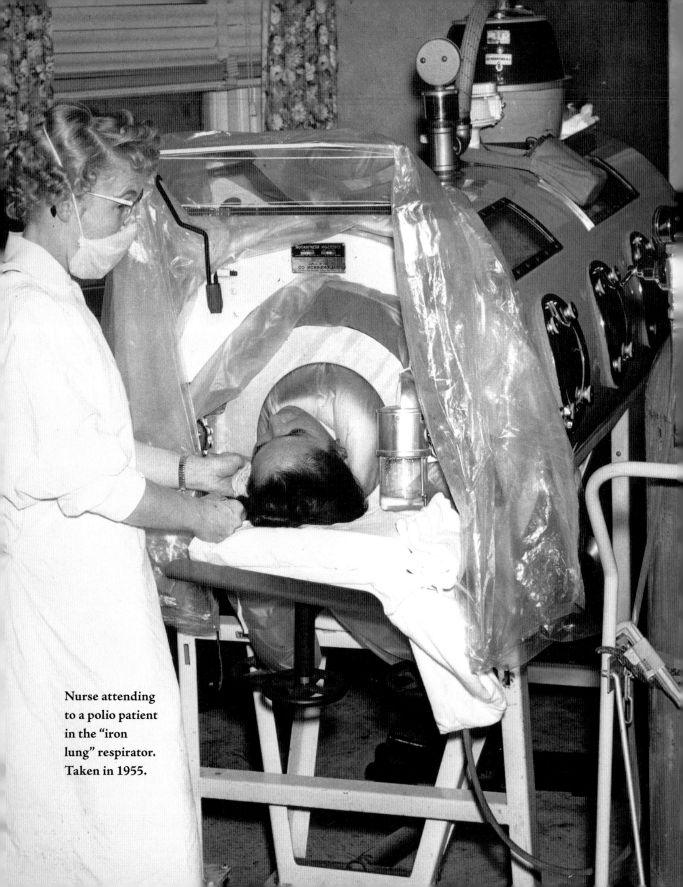

Nurse attending
to a polio patient
in the "iron
lung" respirator.
Taken in 1955.

be a frightening illness that raged nearly every summer and left thousands of people seriously impaired. For those who had dealt with this dreadful disease, it was an extraordinary relief to know that this was the end of respirators, iron lungs, rocking beds, and the horrible crippling effects of the illness.

Croup and Humidifiers

The innovation and ingenuity of the Floating's doctors were not confined to installing air conditioning units. They used these very same traits to make changes to the way they had been managing a persistent pediatric illness.

In the winter months, many of the Floating's youngest patients suffered from laryngotracheobronchitis (croup), a severe respiratory infection. Traditionally, this condition had been treated with warm water vapor therapy, but doctors were increasingly using the more efficacious cold-water vaporization. The Floating had a "vapor room" set up to treat these patients. This was an environment suffused with moisture. The patients were successfully treated, but their beds were soon soaked and it was difficult for the nurses to function in such an atmosphere. The hospital's administrator, Ms. Geneva Katz, decided to see if it could be possible to devise an individual humidified crib unit. Such a crib would provide therapy for one infant at a time and would make it possible to deliver this treatment anywhere in the hospital.

Using materials at hand (a canopy frame, a Burgess tent frame, an ice container, a Walton humidifier stand, and a canopy) she rigged up what she called a "Rube Goldberg contraption." Clumsy as it might have seemed, the new invention worked. Within an hour, the "optimum conditions" were attained. The child received the healing moisture while lying on a soft cotton blanket with another over him. He did not have to be in a wet bed in moist clothing as before.

The new humidification unit also demanded only minor attention from the nurses. Those working with the patients could gain access to them simply by lifting the side of the canopy, lowering the crib side, and letting the canopy fall down over their backs. The transparent canopies made it possible to observe the patients at all times.

Ms. Katz's instructions for setting up these cribs could be easily copied in other hospitals. It is believed her experiment and development of the first portable humidification unit led to the development of the widely used Armstrong Humidifier. [33]

Reverend Rufus Babcock Tobey envisioned the Floating to be a place where poor children could escape the stifling, hot air in Boston's poor neighborhoods.

He may never have imagined the leaps and bounds the hospital would take over the years. Some of those leaps included the surgical advances the doctors of the Floating developed. While they performed minor surgeries on the boat, once the Floating moved to land, their surgical opportunities grew.

In 1945, Dr. Orvar Swenson was appointed as the hospital's first full-time surgeon-in-chief. Dr. Swenson did pioneering work on Hirschsprung's disease, a condition in which a congenital absence of nerves in the lower bowel prevented normal elimination of waste. Children with this disease were forced to depend on enemas. Dr. Swenson's research had led to a surgical method for reconstructing the lower bowel that permitted these children to lead normal lives. He was the only surgeon performing this operation at that time and thus attracted patients from other parts of the country to the Floating, adding to the hospital's financial support. Medical students and other surgeons also came to learn how to perform the surgery.

By the 1960s, the hospital was taking care of children suffering with meningitis, pneumonia, asthma, cancer, leukemia, and the gamut of childhood diseases. Many of the patients in the neonatal unit had undergone newly developed cardiac surgery to repair congenital defects. A four-bed intensive

Ms. Katz's creation: the individual, humidified crib unit. Date unknown.

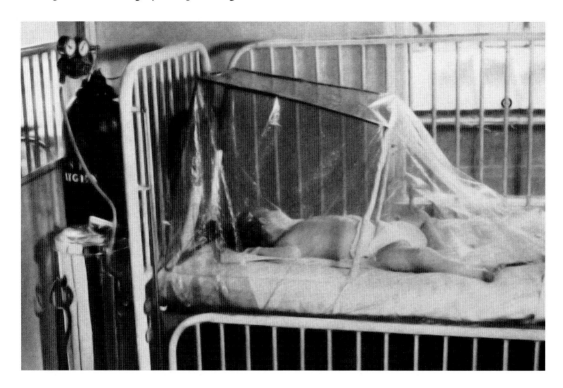

care unit was established on the fifth floor in 1963. Although the Jackson Building had no operating rooms, the pediatric surgeons operated in the adjacent Boston Dispensary on the third floor. On nights and weekends, they shared the adult operating rooms in the Farnsworth Building.

The hospital now performed procedures that Dr. Samuel Breck and other founding doctors would never have imagined. In 1960, Dr. Marshall Kreidberg reported that one hundred infants with hemolytic disease of the newborn, also known as erythroblastosis fetalis, were treated with exchange transfusions every year. This procedure in which the infant's blood is replaced by fresh donor blood through a vein in the umbilical cord was carried out in one small corner of the nursery, just outside the door of the premature nursery. Today, this condition is prevented with an antibody given to pregnant mothers whose fetuses are at risk, and such transfusions are rarely necessary.

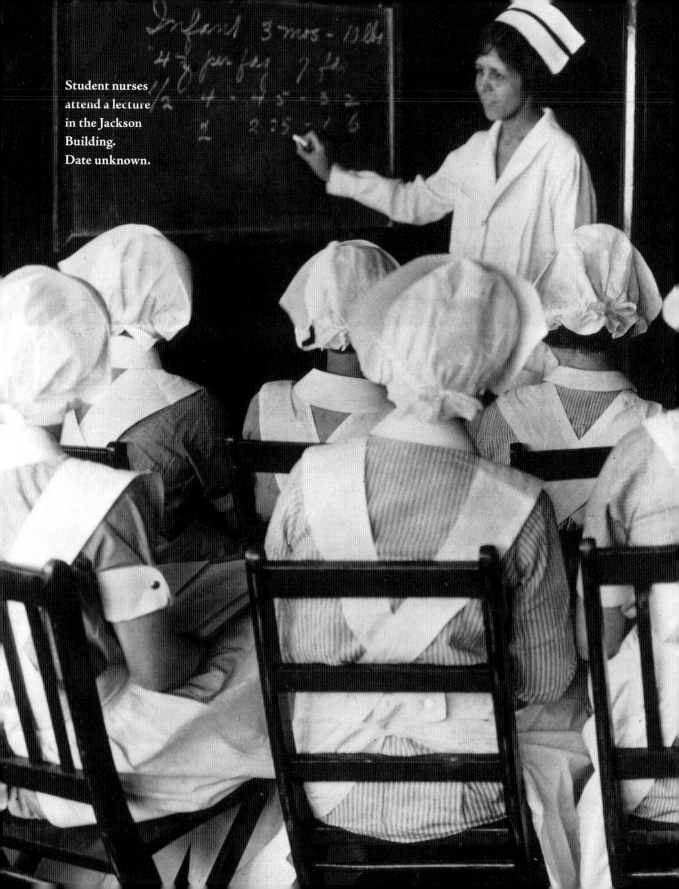

Student nurses
attend a lecture
in the Jackson
Building.
Date unknown.

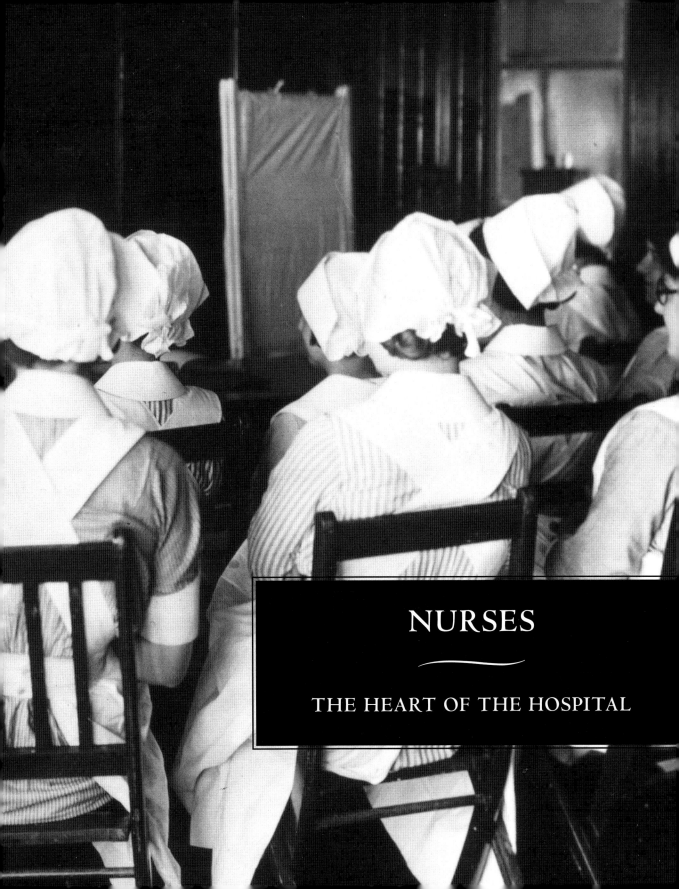

NURSES

THE HEART OF THE HOSPITAL

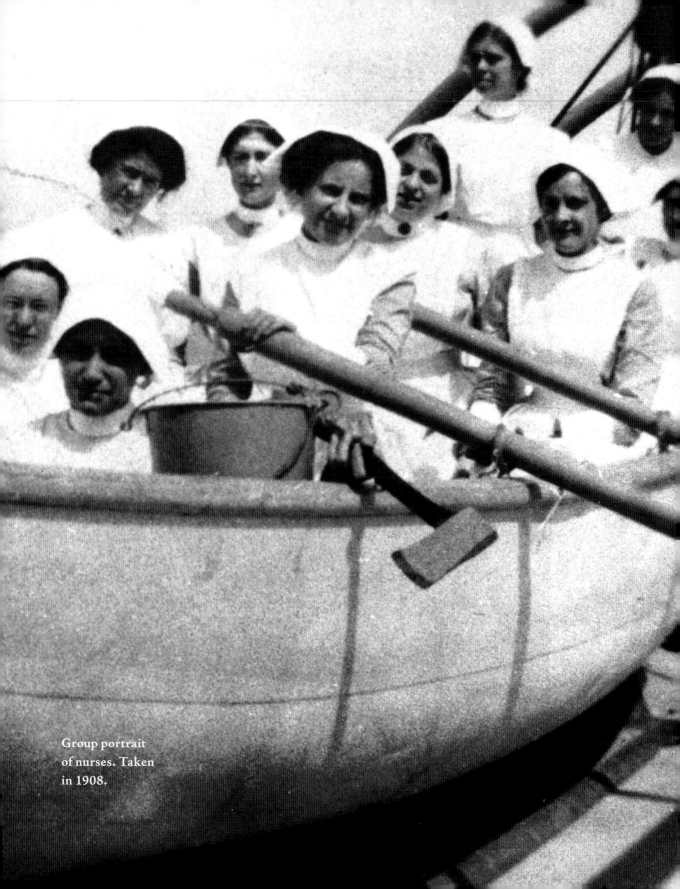

Group portrait of nurses. Taken in 1908.

NURSES

THE HEART OF THE HOSPITAL

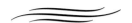

Beginning with the ship's first voyage in 1894, the largest burden of patient care fell on the Floating's thirty nurses. The annual report of 1901 paid tribute to them with the following words: "Few realize the constant attention, the harassing character of the many small details, the infinite amount of patience that must be a part of the nursing of very sick infants. Most of the nurses seriously felt the effect of our short season but harmony and efficiency has characterized the work of the nurses this year as heretofore."[1] By the turn of the twentieth century, all the nurses on The Floating Hospital were graduates of nursing schools, and the volunteers who had given such devoted service were phased out.

Throughout the decades, the nursing staff at the Floating has been the heart and soul of the hospital. Not only are they experts in their fields, the nurses also provide reassurance to frightened children and parents, comforting them with words and kind gestures. Wielding both advanced medical knowledge and a supportive bedside manner, the nurses at the Floating make every child feel special.

Doctors and patients depended on the nursing staff, and in turn, the nursing staff educated themselves so they could provide the best possible care. Graduate nurses were offered a summer course of instruction that included practical work on the wards, in the operating room, and in the food department.[2] The doctors gave lectures on such subjects as the nursing of premature and sickly infants; what to observe in children; therapeutics (drugs); nursing of contagious diseases; the feeding and preparation of modified milk; and many other topics. At the end of each year, graduate nurses received diplomas in the special care of infants. The *American Journal of Nursing*[3] took note of these courses and informed its readers that the Floating offered a graduate program for nurses. The Floating, which had always trained young doctors, had become a full-fledged teaching hospital for both physicians and nurses. The number of nursing graduates rose from eight in 1899 to a peak of fifty in 1914.

In 1909, in the hospital's on-shore facility on East Newton Street, a young woman named Celia Frances Battey attended these lectures and left behind the notebook she kept for her classes. Her notes are hurried transcriptions of the lectures she was hearing, but shed light on the nature of the courses she attended and provide insight into the scientific knowledge that informed the care of patients on board the ship and in the on-shore facility at that time. From her notes, handwritten in pencil, we have a keen and detailed knowledge of the types of instruction nurses obtained and the procedures and practices they conducted at the Floating.

Treating Premature Babies

The Floating took pains to ensure that every child received extensive care, and no one needed this level of attention more than premature babies, defined as those born weighing less than 5½ pounds (2,500 grams) between the twenty-eighth and fortieth week of pregnancy. As late as 1935, the American Academy of Pediatrics defined a premature infant by birth weight, regardless of gestational age.[4] Nurses quickly learned that "intelligent care of [the] nurse may mean life or death to the baby."

When working with premature infants, nurses paid strict attention to the temperatures of the children and their environment, diet, and breathing. Nurses protected these babies from noise, vibrations, and light as much as possible, so that the infants would remain calm enough to eat and breathe normally. In their graduate lectures, nurses learned that the babies' brains were still developing, especially the center of the brain that regulates heat. With this knowledge, they were better equipped to handle these fragile, premature infants.

Nurses who helped deliver premature babies knew to take preventive steps during labor to help both the baby and mother. They prepared cribs that were padded on all four sides with sheets over the top to protect the babies' eyes from the light and warmed the bed with hot water bottles or electric pads. After the babies were born, they didn't bathe or dress them; they had "premature jackets" (cotton wool covered with gauze) ready. These jackets supplied heat while preventing heat loss. They also used gauze pads instead of diapers. The nurses kept premature babies' rooms at a steady 73° to 80° and left the babies alone, without handing or disturbing them too much. They also kept the temperature of the crib at about 80°, knowing that if the cribs became too hot, the infants would die of heat stroke. Only after two or three days did they give the babies baths in warm olive oil. The oil bath cleaned the babies while also providing a massage and preventing heat loss.

This jacket for a premature baby helped the infants regulate their temperatures.

Breck feeder.

The nurses were under strict instructions when it came to feeding these premature babies as well. They knew the mother might not have much breast milk, so they used their best efforts to find her a wet nurse. They usually tried to find someone in the mother's family to help feed the baby. Nurses also stimulated the mother's breasts, so that she would have milk for her baby. If the baby was too weak to nurse, nurses tried a bottle, medicine dropper, Breck feeder, or spoon. The degree to which they diluted the milk with water depended on the baby's weight.

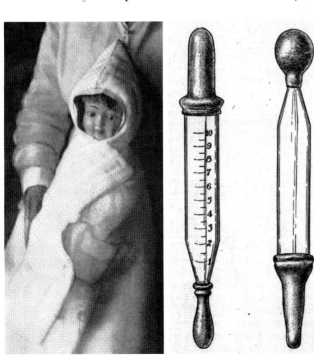

The Floating nurses deftly used the tools they had learned to recognize signs of distress in premature babies. They knew that these infants gained weight slowly and tried to encourage worried mothers. Their support was more than just medical in nature, and their bedside manner assured many anxious mothers.

Skin Diseases

The nurses' work was not limited to caring for newborns; they did much of the care for the majority of diseases on the ship, including ailments of the skin. Nurses learned what to look for when treating these illnesses. The first element of importance was the visual appearance, be it "macule, papule, tubercle, tumor, vesicle, bulla or large vesicle, hives or wheals, crusts, scales, excoriation, fissures, ulcers, or cicatrix scars." The second element of import was the location of the rash, and the third was the configuration, or arrangement, of lesions.

Nurses kept a close eye out for signs of scarlet fever and chicken pox. They treated the latter with a carbolic acid wash and were explicitly instructed not to use "quack medicine," sulphonaphol, carbolic salve, resinol, or mercury. They applied four percent boric acid as a soothing astringent.

When treating children and infants with skin diseases, they often used castile soap, a mild soap with olive oil. For seborrhea, nurses used olive oil and hot water. For eczema, the nurses kept close watch on the children's kidneys and gave them plenty of water. They also tied the children's hands down to keep them from scratching their skin. For eczema, they did not use soap and water, but rather a paste of stearate and talcum powder. Heat rash and hives called for white wash, composed of zinc oxide and glycerine; hives also meant the children received castor oil and lots of water. A more serious condition was impetigo, a contagious infection with pus caused by streptococcus. To treat these crusty vesicles and raw skin, nurses patted the children's face, nose, and scalp with a towel as a moist compress.

Pediculosis (lice) nits were treated with larkspur or a shampoo with crude petroleum every seven days, until the nits no longer hatched. For ringworm of the scalp, nurses applied a carbolic acid solution, made with beta-napthol sulphur and lard, to the scalp every night and washed it out in the morning. Children with scabies received a salve made from benzoin and olive oil in equal parts. The nurses also removed and boiled all clothes that came in contact with the scabies.

Those unfortunate babies who contracted syphilis from their mothers might be born deaf or with a bullous eruption, which could be treated with a 4 percent boric acid wash. Nearly half of all children infected with syphilis during gestation died shortly before or after birth.

The symptoms of syphilitic children usually appeared when the child was four to six weeks old, the most prominent of which was snuffles, due to infection in the nose, with bloody nasal discharge and a hoarse cry from laryngitis. They might show flat, oval, dark brown or red patches on the mouth, anus, hands, or feet, and ulcers on the anus may have a grayish discharge. Later signs included tooth abnormalities, bony changes, neurological involvement, blindness, and deafness.

Syphilis was treated with mercury compounds. Colles' law held that a woman who gave birth to a syphilitic infant could not be infected by the infant she nursed and handled, although any other person was likely to be infected. Mistaken belief in the doctrine of paternal transmission of syphilis was prominent at this time, when in fact the mothers were already infected.

Nurses learned that the spirochete dies in a dry state only after two to three days, so they should not let the children cough in their faces. If nurses were exposed, they used Dobell's solution to rinse out their mouths. If an infected child scratched them, the nurses used castile soap and hot water, or a corrosive if they felt it was necessary. If the nurses were exposed, the doctors instructed them to suck the wound and spit it out and then apply a mercurial ointment immediately.

Nurses who helped deliver syphilitic children cared for the children full time, as these newborns were not allowed to go home with their mothers. The fate of these poor children is unknown. They were either sent to orphanages or spent their too-short lives on the boat.

Infectious Diseases

Like many of its contemporaries, the Floating took special care to fight infection and pathogens. Nurses were familiar with reading bacterial cultures and stool samples, as well as how to recognize safe and unsafe bacteria, be it through lab results or their senses of smell.

The lectures taught nurses that scarlet fever comes on suddenly, sometimes with a headache and vomiting. While children did not usually report a sore throat, nurses could easily recognize the rash that started on the chest and back and spread upward and downward, lasting six or seven days. They made sure the doctor made his diagnosis during this first stage, before sepsis in the throat or cardiac complications appeared. They treated the patient with hygienic care and a low-protein diet that aimed to save the kidneys. Children received plenty of water, bed rest, and help in eliminating their bowels with a saline cathartic (not with calomel [mercury chloride]). Nurses gave children with scarlet fever a warm bath each day in hope of preventing nephritis and uremia. Sometimes, they administered strychnine or iron during convalescence, but usually the children received very few drugs. Children with scarlet fever stayed in the hospital for anywhere from seven weeks to three months or more.

Measles was much more contagious than scarlet fever. It presented with a blotchy red rash and fever. Due to the highly contagious nature of measles, nurses made their diagnosis during the acute stage. They treated children with hygienic fresh air and sunshine. If children developed ulcers in their corneas, nurses washed out their eyes with a boric acid solution. If there was severe inflammation, nurses used argyrols antiseptic, containing 20 percent silver, or ice compresses. The children received plenty of water, lemonade, and saffron tea.

Diphtheria was a particular concern for nurses. It was highly contagious, and though a case might be mild, it could persist for months. Nurses recognized it by the characteristic membrane swelling in the throat and discharge from the nose. They treated this insidious disease quickly with antitoxins. Untreated, diphtheria could lead to complications such as paralysis and heart failure.

For children with infantile paralysis (polio), nurses could recognize the telltale signs of fever, digestive disturbance, and then muscular paralysis. The medical community knew little of this potentially fatal disease: it was known that polio was contagious, but doctors were not sure how it was spread, although the horsefly was suspected. If the nurses saw an infant who contracted this disease, they disinfected the baby's throat and cleaned out his intestinal tract.

Cleft Palate

The Floating nurses were experts in dealing with the challenges presented by birth deformities, such as cleft palate. They knew how cleft palates presented, what complications might occur, and when a child would be ready for the corrective surgery.

Before the surgery, it fell to the nurses to care for the infants, make sure they were getting enough food, and avoid the complications that resulted from a cleft palate. They helped mothers nurse these infants and made sure they did not develop any digestion problems. If the babies did get diarrheal disease, the nurses ensured they got enough breast milk for the disease to pass.

With a cleft palate, there is nothing that prevents the food from passing into the nose, which might cause infection. When caring for these infants, nurses kept the nose and mouth clean and washed out the babies' mouths with a boric acid solution to prevent infection after they had milk.

After the corrective surgery, which was done anywhere from birth to seven years of age, but usually when the child was around eighteen months old, the child's recovery was left in the nurses' hands. They ensured that the children did not disrupt the stitches by keeping them calm with morphine or bromide. Instead of using a bottle, they fed children with a sterilized medicine dropper, Breck feeder, or spoon. They never forced the mouth open with a tongue depressor to check how the palate was healing. Instead, they used a stitch of silk through the tongue to pull it forward and check the mouth.

Spina Bifida

Nurses were also skilled in helping patients recover from spina bifida surgery. Babies who suffered from spina bifida underwent surgery just days after birth. After the surgery, nurses took pains to keep the area completely clean with the babies lying on their faces with their buttocks up in the air. They sealed the wound with gauze and collodion. They also put strips of adhesive on the buttocks across from the wound to keep urine and stool from entering the wound.

Surgical Care

Not only did nurses become experts in the care of infants and children who needed surgery, they were familiar with the operations as well. Ms. Battey's notes include detailed explanations and diagrams of surgeries to correct intussusception, umbilical hernias, femoral hernias, and appendicitis. Nursing students were familiar with tracheotomy intubations and learned how to drain the mastoid cells behind a child's ears. Nurses knew to treat tuberculosis of the bones with food, fresh air, and rest, and they also knew that, following surgery, children needed more than just basic treatment to help them deal with the disease. To relieve weight from their upper bodies, nurses put children on their backs on a Bradford frame or in braces and plaster jackets.

Clubbed Foot

The nurses were also responsible for caring for children with clubbed feet. These deformities are a result of a cramped position in the uterus, but could be corrected as soon as the pressure was relieved. To help these babies, nurses bent the foot into shape whenever they were near the babies' bedsides. They redistributed the balance of the muscles and reshaped the bones. Since the condition was liable to relapse, one could overcorrect the foot by stretching it in a plaster cast.

Diseases of the Mind

Nurses at the Floating made sure that every child was treated with love and respect. When they treated mentally deficient ("backward") children, they never referred to them as "imbeciles" or "idiots," as was common at the time. They knew that if properly trained, some of these children might overcome their deficiencies. These children may have been born of alcoholic women or parents with epilepsy. They may have exhibited reduced vitality due to tuberculosis, rheumatism, or gout. If the mother was weak or ill, the child's chances of being strong mentally and/or physically were reduced as well.

Nurses could quickly recognize symptoms of mentally deficient children, and they watched carefully for developmental milestones, such as smiling, sitting, and walking by certain ages.

In 1910, Ms. Battey received her Graduate Nursing Diploma and went on to work at the Hospital for Women and Children in Syracuse, New York.

> After a strenuous day spent in constant attendance at the bedsides of very sick infants, many nurses had a long trolley or railroad ride home. By the turn of the century, the Floating found a solution to their long commutes. The twenty-three nurses on Ms. L.A. Wilber's staff lived at the Maverick House in East Boston and were "boarded" (had their meals) on the hospital ship.

THE HEART OF THE HOSPITAL

After the Floating moved to the Jackson Building at 20 Ash Street in 1931, the staff found it antiquated and crowded, and they often had a hard time coping with the lack of amenities. Despite the accommodations, the atmosphere was friendly and informal, and the professional services met the highest standards.

At first, the nurses wore uniforms, but they soon gave up wearing their caps partly because they got in the way when a nurse had to bend down over a crib or take care of a patient in a bed surrounded by equipment. In the early

1970s, after the families of patients expressed a preference for a less institutional approach, uniforms disappeared altogether. Nurses were assigned their own patients, and it was generally believed the continuity of care made the children feel more at home. The nurse soon became a friend instead of a stranger. The doctors were vital, of course, but they were not always there. Nurses were a constant that the children could count on and someone the parents could trust and talk to.

Everything was done to make the Floating's still-cramped quarters efficient from a medical standpoint while creating a non-threatening, cheerful atmosphere for the patients and their parents. The hospital staff was always looking for new ways to make the time a child spent in the hospital more pleasant. For instance, the food for the Floating, cooked in the diet kitchens at the Dispensary, was at first geared to adult tastes, and most of the meals didn't appeal to children. When the plates kept coming back barely touched, Ms. Geneva Katz, the hospital's administrator, modified the menu to include hamburgers and hot dogs, and appetites improved.

The nurses gave medications and took temperatures, but they also made popcorn and threw parties for the patients. At one of the annual Fourth of July roof deck picnics, a member of the house staff pushed a piano onto the elevator, and there was music on the roof. Halloween was another big day, and parents were encouraged to bring costumes for their children.

Nurses sometimes bent the rules for the patients who were very ill. Several nurses who worked at the Floating during the 1970s reminisced about their work and recalled the time a desperately ill child wanted to see his dog. The nurses remembered how wonderful it was to see the look on the boy's face as his lively little dog bounded into the room. They also remembered another very sick boy who had always wanted to see a copy of *Playboy Magazine*. This, too, was managed. "These kids were like our own," one of the nurses said. "We all became like one large family."

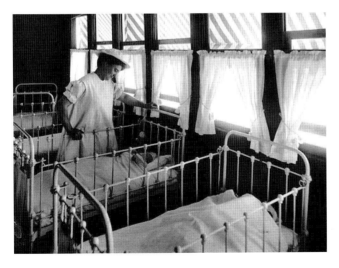

A nurse looking over her patients. Taken in 1909.

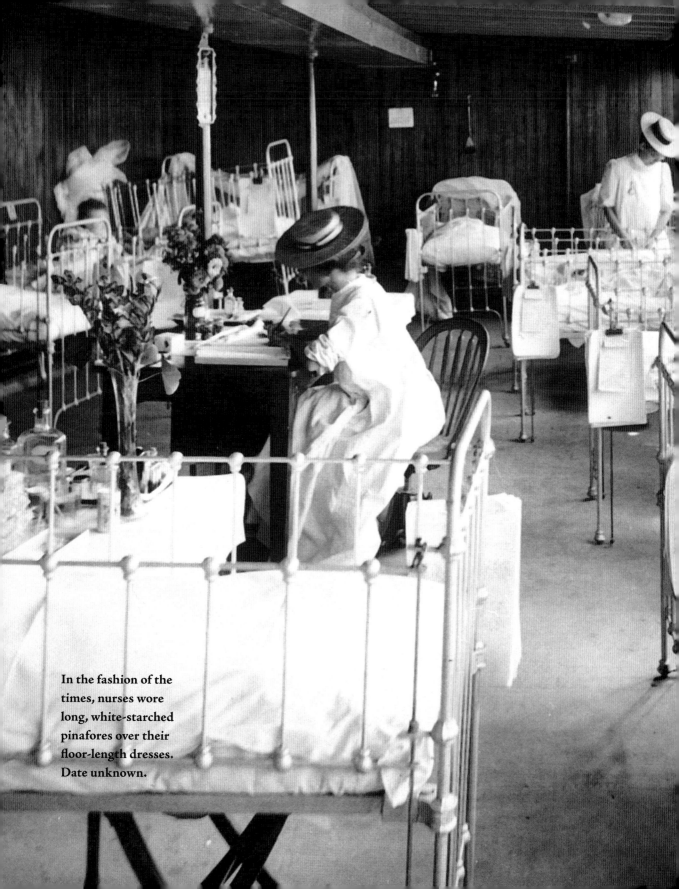

In the fashion of the times, nurses wore long, white-starched pinafores over their floor-length dresses. Date unknown.

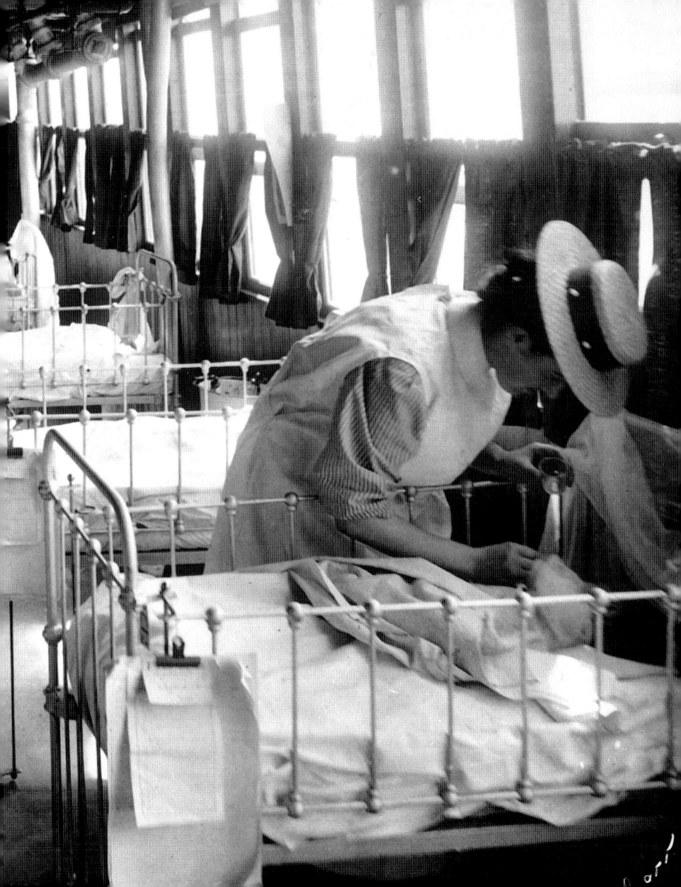

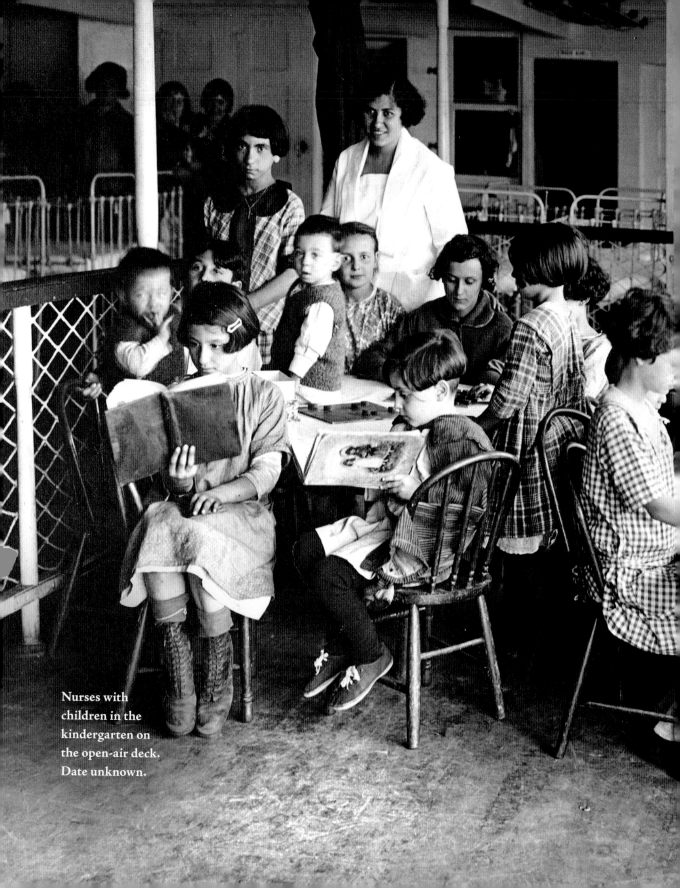

Nurses with children in the kindergarten on the open-air deck. Date unknown.

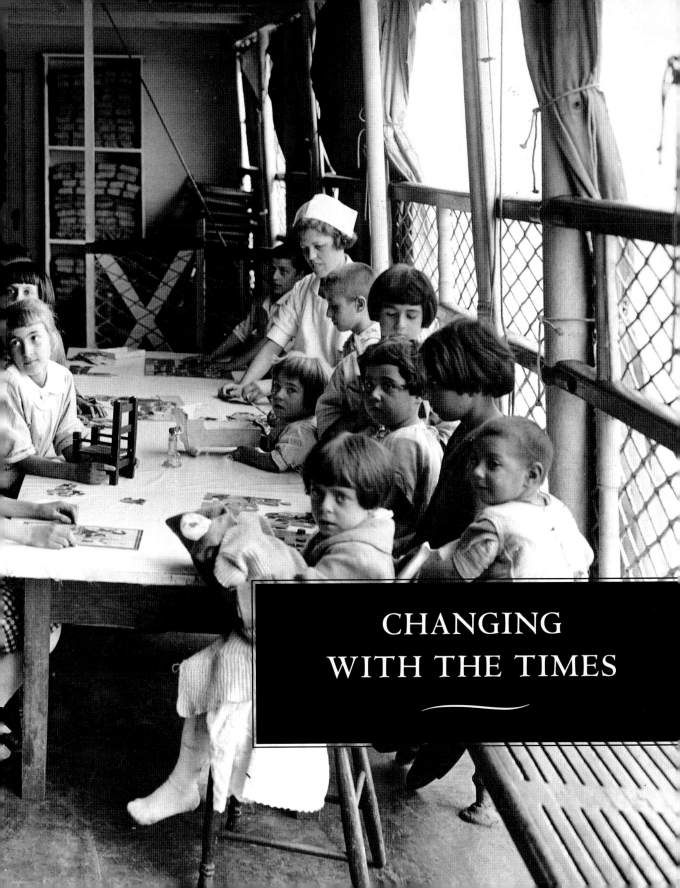

CHANGING
WITH THE TIMES

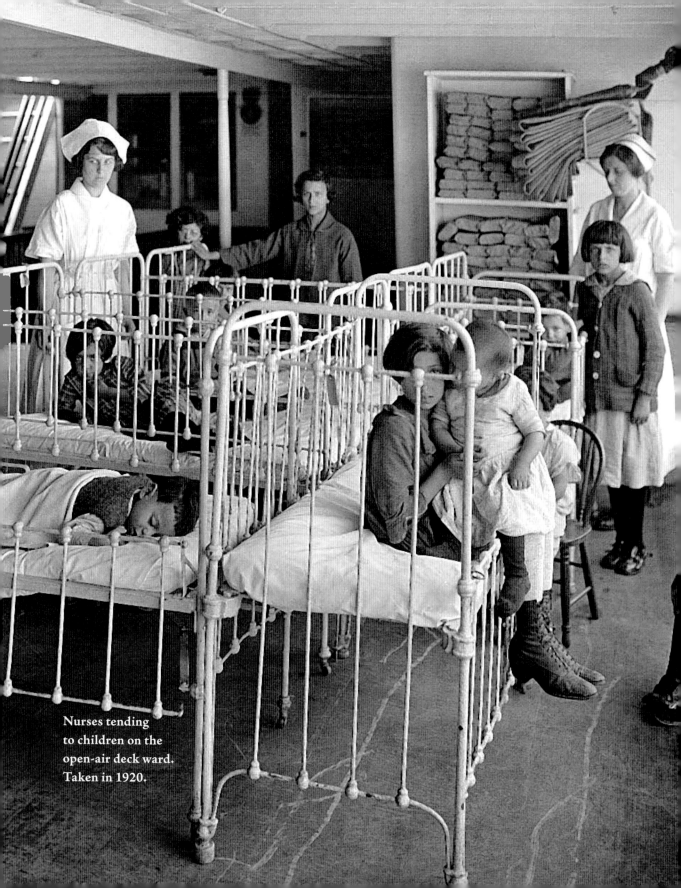

Nurses tending to children on the open-air deck ward. Taken in 1920.

CHANGING WITH THE TIMES

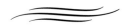

Nearly a decade after its first journey and modest beginnings, almost two hundred fifty doctors[1] had sent patients to the Floating. The hospital had established a good working relationship with The Infants' Hospital, Children's Hospital, Carney Hospital, Fayette Street Dispensary, and the outpatient departments of the Boston City Hospital and Massachusetts General Hospital. At the end of each season, several of these institutions accepted patients who were declared still too sick to go home. The hospital's reputation, prominence, and prestige attracted poor families from all over New England.

The new ship also meant many changes within the Floating. The men and women so integral in founding the hospital were slowly passing the baton to the next generation of leaders. The Floating's services were expanding to shore as well. The on-shore clinic saw patients all year, providing the children of Boston valuable services when it was too cold for the Floating to go into the harbor. The biggest change, however, came about in a most unfortunate way. A devastating fire in 1927 changed the Floating forever.

ON-SHORE DEPARTMENT

The Floating's work was never confined to the boat. From its inception, nurses would visit patients in their homes; they knew their work did not end once the children left the ship. Soon after the turn of the twentieth century, the Floating's staff realized that they needed to formally expand their services during the cooler months.

In 1911, the annual report summed up the accomplishments of the hospital:

"From a quest for health to be found in the breezes of the harbor for a few children to a hospital caring for thousands suffering from every disease peculiar to childhood as well as many of those common to mankind; from a hired barge to a hospital equipped to care of more children than any other in the country; from a few volunteer care-takers locally interested to a corps of graduate nurses of country-wide selection, including often superintendents of other hospitals; from graduate nurses giving of their training, to graduate nurses sent to all parts of our country with an experience not offered elsewhere; from the purchase of an anchor that the boat may be kept in mid-stream through the night in the endeavor to save two lives to twenty-four hour service throughout the summer and a night anchorage—these are some of the progressive steps taken. Each has been in response to a legitimate demand, and the meeting of the demand has opened a new possibility.

A more stable "hurricane deck" provides the sun's healing rays for twelve months of the year, whenever the weather is suitable. Date unknown.

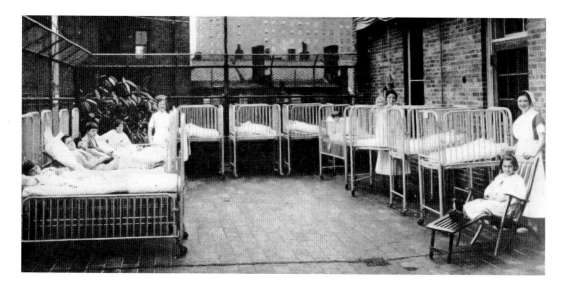

And so has come the development of our On Shore work, which during its third year has occupied the time of two visitors. Plans have already been made for the extension of this work in 1912, whereby its benefits may be carried to those who may not come in direct contact with the work on the boat."[2]

The last sentences of that paragraph refer to the program that had sent nurses to visit patients in their homes almost since the first season of the hospital. This aspect of the Floating's mission was becoming equally important to its work during the summer on board the boat. The outreach program continued to grow, and in 1916, the permanent on-shore department of the Floating was established in the Norfolk House Center on John Eliot Square in Roxbury, a building housing several charities.[3]

With the establishment of the on-shore department, the hospital was transformed from a seasonal health care facility into a year-round health care provider. Resident physicians and nurses were on duty at Norfolk House to serve patients who had been on board during the summer, as well as patients who had never set foot on the ship. Former patients were given check-ups, and new patients were examined and treated if sick or referred to other hospitals if they needed inpatient care. Children from all over the city were welcome. Home visitation was directed from the on-shore department, which helped with record keeping and follow up. Of course, there was no charge for this service, even though it added to the Floating's expenses.

With America's entry into World War I, the work continued, but publication of the hospital's annual reports was curtailed or abbreviated to save paper. The on-shore clinics were flourishing, and research continued. Due to the wartime shortage of doctors, Dr. Eli Friedman, the resident physician, had to share his time with another hospital. During the winter of 1918, the Floating was pressed into service as a dormitory for sailors. The USS *Boston Floating Hospital* was commissioned by the U.S. Navy on January 7, 1918, and returned to her owner on June 2, 1918. When the Navy returned the boat, the hospital had been largely restored to its former condition but needed some repairs.[4]

The pediatricians on shore were also kept busy treating infectious diseases such as measles, scarlet fever, diphtheria, and whooping cough. There were twenty-six deaths in 1922[5] among the children who were seen at the clinics with such illnesses, but children with these diseases were still not seen on the Floating boat. Furthermore, the on-shore clinic and other Boston hospitals informed the Floating about the presence of communicable diseases in a family or immediate neighborhood so that the hospital could be on the lookout for symptoms and protect the babies in the wards against such illnesses.

During the Floating's 1926 season, there was an unexplained increase in the kind of severe gastroenteric diseases that had led to the hospital's founding. The mortality rate from intestinal infections was high that summer (out of 235 permanent patients and 319 day patients, 12.3 percent died), and five patients died within forty-eight hours of admission. The intestinal problems were treated with the intravenous administration of fluids, and blood transfusions were given to almost all these patients so that they would have "normal blood" with which to combat the infection.[6]

On board, the hospital set up special clinics for cardiac cases, for those with postural and nutritional defects, and for patients who were thought to need heliotherapy, or exposure to sunlight, because of rickets or other orthopedic defects.

FIRE

At the end of the summer of 1926, the Floating was towed to the Atlantic Works shipyard in East Boston so that it could be refurbished for the next season. A bond issue (5 percent, ten-year gold debentures) raised the fifty thousand dollars needed to replace the engines and boilers from Mrs. L.G. Burnham's yacht after two decades of hard wear. Once the maintenance work was completed, the ship was towed across the harbor to its dock at the North End Pier, ready to set out to sea for the 1927 season.

During the evening of June 1, 1927, Captain Grover was awakened by smoke in his cabin.[7] He quickly turned on the boat's fire alarm to alert the others. Captain Grover could see that the pier was on fire, and so he jumped into the water. Two members of the crew, Eliot Myrick and Ralph Renshaw, and watchman Lawrence Penny were asleep on the children's upper deck. The three men launched a lifeboat because one of them couldn't swim. All made it to shore unhurt.

On shore, Patrolman Michael J. Rizzo of the Hanover Station in the North End was clearing the North End Pier, a notorious trysting place of "spooners." He had just scared off several young couples when he chanced to look over his shoulder and saw a "flicker of flame" on the pier.

Within seconds, the flames spread to the boat. His call to the fire department resulted in four alarms. The first was at 11:22 p.m., the last at 11:31 p.m.

So quickly were they sounded that it seemed as if there was one long steady blast from the tapper.

Engine 47, one of the city's fireboats, had just been equipped with its first radio. It was on an island in the harbor answering what turned out to be a false alarm when the radio summoned it to the North End Pier. Engine 47 joined other fire boats and on-shore efforts that were trying to extinguish the blaze, but the flames spread so quickly there was obviously no hope of saving the boat. When the fire was finally extinguished, the steel hull was all that was left.

It was a spectacular blaze, and automobiles from all over the area were attracted to Commercial Street by the sight of smoke and flames. It seemed as if the entire population of the North End had turned out to see the fire. The glare could be seen in Salem, fifteen miles north, and the fire burned so long that a Salem resident was able to drive to the pier in time to see the spectacle at its height. The newspaper accounts report that the entire harbor—from Charlestown Bridge to East Boston to the South Shore—was as light as day, and smoke hung over the South Shore towns of Hingham and Cohasset well after midnight. During the early morning hours and into the day, the streets were filled with people and automobiles gawking at the spectacle.

G. Loring Briggs, the hospital's manager, was at home in Brookline when the *Boston Globe* called to inform him about what had happened. Mr. Briggs' son drove him to the harbor where, after a time, he was reassured that no one had been injured. The boat, however, had burned down to the water line.

Mrs. Filena Steward Robinson had been a student nurse on the

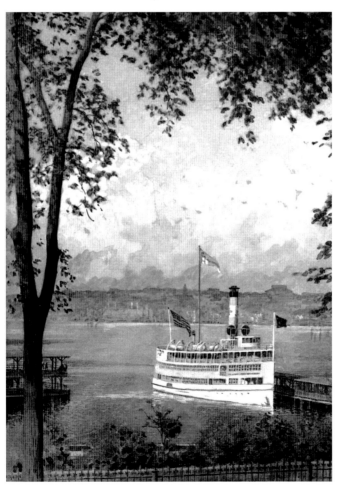

The Floating, just before sailing for the night anchorage. It is moored at the North End Pier as seen from Copp's Hill Burying Ground. Taken in 1908.

Floating in 1926. When the boat caught fire, she was a district nurse at the Hull Street Medical Mission in the North End. Mrs. Robinson later recalled that she was at work in the Mission waiting for "the evening rush" of patients when she looked across the cemetery in front of the Mission and saw the boat aflame. It had been known for some time that the usefulness of the boat was diminishing because the patients on board now had mild diseases and those with more serious illnesses were now treated at other hospitals. However, Mrs. Robinson said, the feeling of all who knew the boat was that it was a terrible loss.[8]

With amazing foresight, Ralph Lowell, treasurer of the Floating, had been instrumental in convincing a reluctant board of directors to take out a two-hundred-thousand-dollar fire insurance policy on the boat in 1926. The boat had been valued at one hundred fifty thousand dollars before the end of what turned out to be its last season, but when the fire destroyed it, the new boilers had already been installed, raising its value to two hundred thousand dollars.

In December 1932, General Ship & Engine Works was asked to convert the burned-out hull of the old Boston Floating Hospital into a coastal oil tanker. In 1933, the ship was relaunched as a 675-gross-ton diesel-powered tanker named *Marshall B. Hall*. It was disposed of in 1952.[9] It was generally agreed that the boat had served its purpose. It was time to retire it and move on shore.

MAJOR CONTRIBUTORS

The boat's time had come to an end, and the board of directors began to plan for a permanent building on land. For these on-shore plans to be realized, the Floating would have to raise the money to finance a brand-new building. The two hundred thousand dollars from the insurance policy was not enough to build the new hospital, so the trustees began to look elsewhere. A large portion of what was needed was found in the estate of two brothers named Jackson.

Paul Wilde Jackson had died in 1928, leaving an estate of more than four hundred thousand dollars. His legacy also included that of his late brother, Henry Clay Jackson, whose will had been unsigned. Henry Jackson was a force behind the development of the West End Street Railway Company, the forerunner of the Boston Elevated and Massachusetts Bay Transportation Authority (MBTA), and his will included a trust fund designed to benefit the families of Boston Transit Company employees.

Mr. Lowell, who was also a trustee of the Jackson Trust, was instrumental in convincing his fellow trustees to contribute two hundred thousand dollars of its assets to the construction of the new building of the Floating. "According to my recollection," said Henry Brainerd, a New England Medical Center trustee, "the thinking was that there could be no better memorial to the Jackson brothers than to build the hospital, name the main building after them, and provide care not only for the children of the Transit employees but to all other children of Boston." [10] The Jackson Building was completed in 1931.

CHANGES IN LEADERSHIP

The launch of a new boat in 1906 meant more patients, and as the patient load became larger, so did the team of hospital leaders. Dr. Samuel Breck continued as chairman of the visiting staff; Dr. C.D. Wilkins became medical superintendent; Henry G. Megathlin was general superintendent; and John R. Anderson, the hospital's first superintendent, became assistant manager. Over the years, Mr. Anderson had served as a contact between the hospital's administration and potential contributors. [11]

Mr. Anderson was well known around Boston as "the eloquent and effective Scotch Temperance Orator." In a brochure promoting his appearances, he was called an "up-to-date speaker, one who is not constantly threshing over old straw but who keeps pace with the times and brings new thoughts and fresh illustrations to his addresses." [12] Temperance audiences were interested in the Floating because, like so many others imbued with the spirit of Protestant ethics in those days, they blamed excessive drinking for many of the ills of society and considered the outlawing of drink a method of social reform. Drinking led to family abuse and exacerbated poverty and, by extension, could lead to disease.

Mr. Anderson brought news about the Floating to temperance meetings and recruited support from "pulpit and platform in every section of Massachusetts. Mr. Anderson never declines an invitation to visit any community or locality manifesting a desire to obtain information relative to the hospital, its object, methods, management and conditions. By no other possible means could the constituencies reached by Mr. Anderson be so effectively enlightened and stirred to sympathy with regard to The Boston Floating Hospital as is the result of his efforts." [13]

Mr. Briggs became the business manager of the Floating in 1906, and his experience in business was an enormous asset to the hospital's fundraising efforts and the organization of its finances. He served as manager until 1927.

In 1906, Edward R. Warren succeeded Reverend Tobey as board chairman. Mr. Warren served in that post until 1912. After his retirement from the Floating, Reverend Tobey continued to support good works from his office at 45 Milk Street, where he oversaw several charities. The Memorial Trust, which he founded, was devoted to charity work soliciting donations from relatives and friends of those who had died. These were "funds that otherwise the relative would have spent to build a monument." The fund's motto was that "lives once useful could be useful again." Reverend Tobey also founded the Ingleside, a residential school for girls who "without school might have led destructive lives." He was an officer of the Howard Benevolent Society, which distributed food to needy families, and he was vice president of the Mount Pleasant Home for aged men and women. [14]

Reverend Tobey continued to be listed in the Floating's annual reports as "Founder of the Hospital" long after he was no longer active in the institution. He died in Middleborough, Massachusetts, on January 6, 1920, of arteriosclerosis at the age of seventy. An obituary tribute in *The Congregationalist* summed up Reverend Tobey's life and his philosophy: [15]

"He was best known as the founder of the Boston Floating Hospital, a charity for sick babies, which he established while he was associate pastor of Berkeley Temple and carried on philanthropic measures whose results were seen far and wide. He loved the individual 'case.' His was not a mere scientific interest in the problem of charity, but a deep-going affection for the visitations of poverty, suffering and human injustice. He will be remembered and blessed for years to come, in many a home which he has brightened and restored, by many a life which he put on its feet after it had stumbled or fallen."

At his death, Reverend Tobey's second wife, Genevieve, survived him, as did his daughter, Mrs. Avis T. Johnson of Middleborough.

Reverend Tobey's death was not the Floating's only loss. Dr. Henry Ingersoll Bowditch, who was instrumental in many of the medical breakthroughs described earlier, resigned from the hospital in 1924 due to ill health and died on June 8, 1926. An extremely personal tribute was contained in a letter of eulogy written by an unnamed but "famous" pediatrician. The author vividly expressed the way many people felt about Dr. Bowditch: [16]

"When an ordinary man dies, his friends are grieved at the time, and then things go on about the same. Once in a while there occurs a rare spirit of such beauty and radiance that the loss is greater and more permanent. Harry was such a spirit; the kindly touch of his hand, the obvious good will and friendliness that shone in his smile, marked him as a man entirely apart from the ordinary. Dr. John Lovett Morse said to me not long ago that by his untiring enthusiasm, originality and unselfishness he had done more for pediatrics than any man in Boston and ... The Boston Floating Hospital is and will continue to be a lasting monument to him ... His greatest achievement was himself; to show other men that even in this day of careless selfishness and disregard for spirituality, a spiritual and Christ-like life could be led and a little of it, I hope, has gone out into each one of us who loved him."

Dr. Paul W. Emerson, who served for a year, succeeded Dr. Bowditch. Dr. Lawrence W. Smith succeeded Dr. Emerson in 1925.

LOVE ON DECK

During the 1920s, college students were given summer jobs on the Floating Hospital. They helped in the kitchen, washed lab equipment, and did other non-medical work on board. One of those students was Libby Dana. She was living in Florida in 1994 when she recalled her summer on the Floating Hospital in a letter she wrote to the author of this history:

"In 1922, I was a freshman at Jackson-Tufts University. At that time the Boston Board of Education had an office where college students, who needed summer jobs, could apply. I made an appointment and was delighted to learn that they had an opening at The Boston Floating Hospital. The secretary said, rather hesitatingly, 'You'll have to be on board at 6 a.m.' I said, 'That's OK.' The next day I had an interview with the steward. When I boarded the ship I was faced with two staircases, one up, one down. Then, lucky me, a young man came down the stairs. I said, 'I wonder if you could direct me to the steward's office.' He said, 'I'll take you there.'

"The job was very simple. Serve the medical interns meals, family style, desserts and coffee or tea individually. Check in at 6 a.m. The boat docked back home at 3 p.m. We also took turns taking the linen tablecloths and napkins to the laundry. When it was my turn I opened the door and a voice said, 'May I carry that for you?' It was my handsome guide of a few days ago.

"During my free time, I used to sit on deck trying to do my summer reading, as far away as possible, from the other five waitresses, giggling and gossiping about the good-looking interns on board. Occasionally I would hear footsteps passing but, being shy at 18, I carefully kept my eyes glued to the page, though I knew it was my handsome guide. After a week of peek-a-boo, I looked up and smiled. He came right over. He was a sophomore at Harvard. We were both 'peace activists' before the phrase was coined.

"It was 'love at first sight' which blossomed into 50 glorious years of harmonious marriage. [Her husband became an expert in large scale feeding and a consultant in kitchen planning for large hotels and the Air Force Academy.] For our 50th anniversary our daughter and son surprised us with a celebration at (the Boston waterfront restaurant) Anthony's Pier 4 'where it all began.'

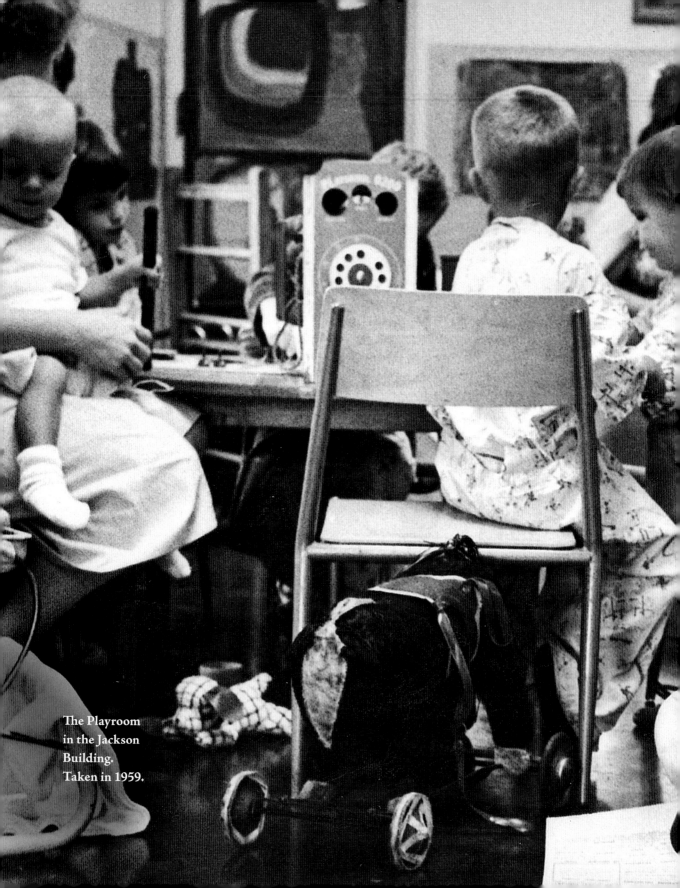

The Playroom
in the Jackson
Building.
Taken in 1959.

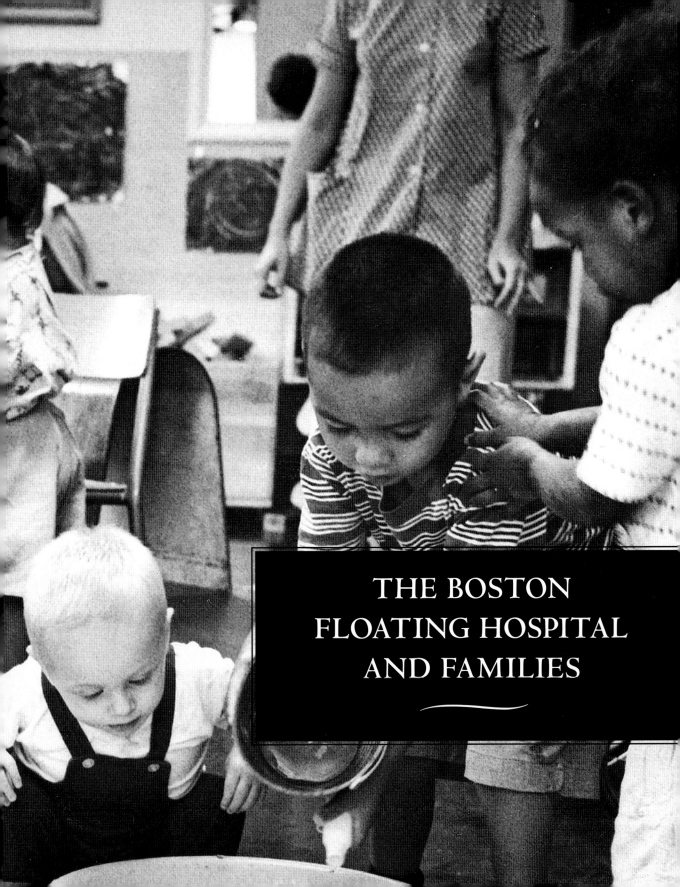

THE BOSTON
FLOATING HOSPITAL
AND FAMILIES

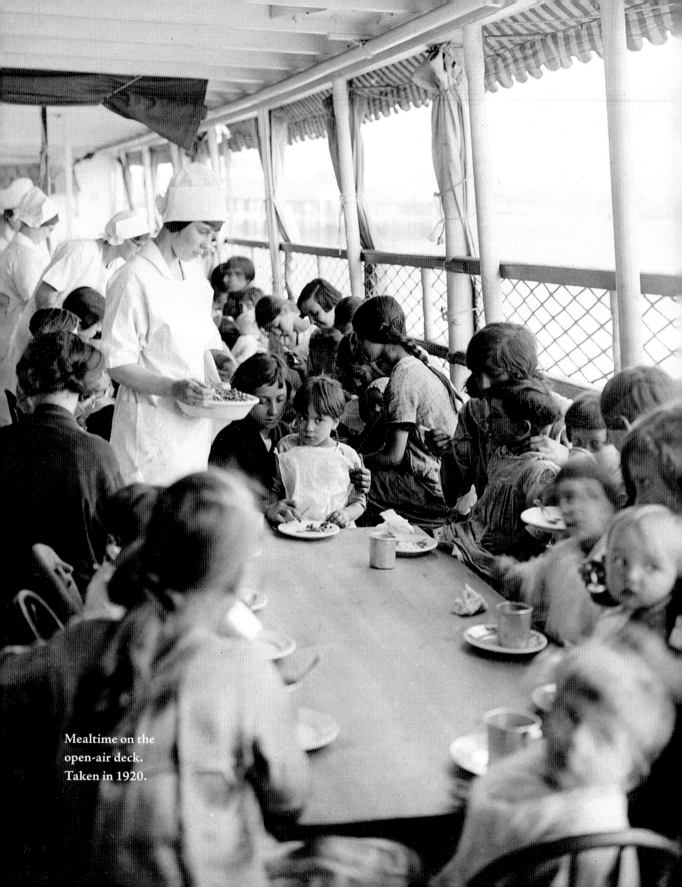

Mealtime on the
open-air deck.
Taken in 1920.

THE BOSTON FLOATING HOSPITAL
AND FAMILIES

One of the hallmarks of the Floating's mandate was to educate families in the treatment of their children. Indeed, the Floating was a pioneer in parent education and placed a previously unheard of importance on the collaboration between families and health care providers. Not only did this part of the mandate never change, it became stronger as the decades rolled by. Visitors are often surprised to find real beds in the hospital rooms. Provided so that parents of sick children can spend the night comfortably, these beds are reminiscent of the welcoming nature of the doctors and nurses on the *Clifford* in 1894. While medical innovations advanced by leaps and bounds, some things never changed.

The loving and nurturing atmosphere of the boat also strengthened over the years. Evidence of this environment can be seen in the Floating's famous playroom.

THE PLAYROOM

The Boston Floating Hospital playroom in the Jackson Building was the first such program in Boston and only the tenth in the country. It was launched under the supervision of the Department of Psychiatry's Child Guidance Unit, and its staff included psychologists, social workers, play therapists, experienced teachers, and a group of assistants and volunteers. On some level, every child in the hospital was involved in its activities.[1] When it was first introduced, the supervisors were Dr. Veronica B. Tisza, the hospital's chief child psychiatrist, and Dr. Rowland Freedman, chief of psychiatry. Mrs. Kristine Angoff ran the playroom from 1948 to 1987. Under her guidance, it became a model for the many similar programs that would be established throughout the country.

The playroom was open all day on weekdays and until noon on Saturdays. Every child permitted to leave his or her hospital bed was welcome in the playroom, a large, airy double room, decorated with plants and pictures. One section was equipped with small tables and chairs and all sorts of toys and games for younger children. On the other side, older children found a punching bag, games and puzzles, and adult-size furniture. The hospital provided the children with every kind of arts and crafts material—crayons, paints, finger paints, as well as a phonograph, games, and jigsaw puzzles. There was stiff competition for the real fireman's hat donated by the Boston Fire Department. The list of articles found in the playroom reads like the inventory of a large toy store.

On one end of the room, there was a one-way mirror through which psychiatrists and psychologists could observe the children at play. Mrs. Angoff encouraged the physicians to come into the playroom so that they could be in direct contact with the children. The room had a Dutch door that made it easy for the staff to see what their patients were doing and to interact with them in a positive manner. In this way, they were often able to help children who seemed to be having problems. And those patients who displayed emotional difficulties were involved in play therapy to help them come to terms with their problems and to help the doctors diagnose the nature of the difficulties.

Everyone who worked in the playroom was aware of the medical condition of each child. Although to the children it functioned as a place of recreation and fun, the playroom had multiple goals: to study the effects of hospitalization on the child, to help spot and ameliorate problems, and to make the hospital stay more pleasant by minimizing the traumatic effects of hospitalization on the

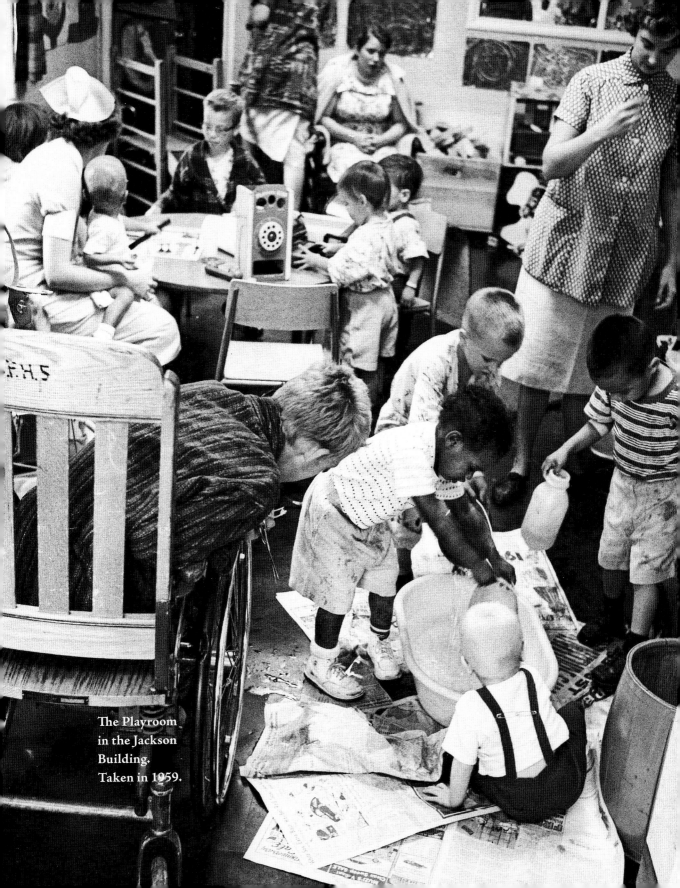

The Playroom
in the Jackson
Building.
Taken in 1959.

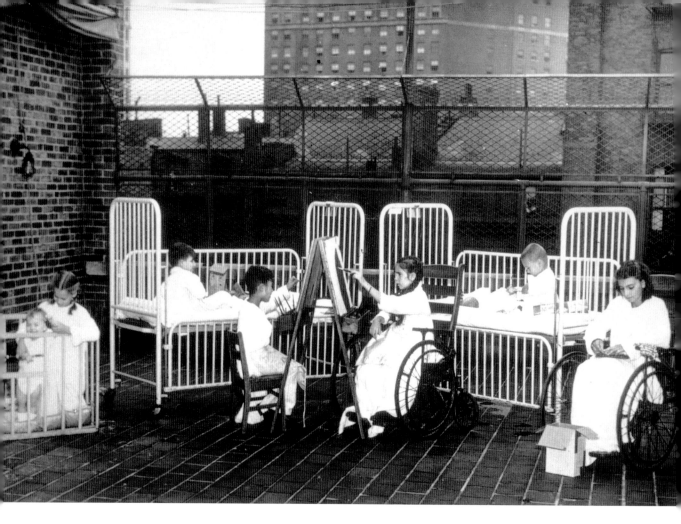

child. The trained staff was always alert for children who exhibited symptoms of psychological difficulties or who had trouble adjusting to their hospital stay.

At least once a morning, a playroom teacher visited those children confined to bed with a toy cart piled high with every imaginable plaything. Rattles and soft balls were given to the littlest babies; color stacks and squeaky rubber animals were available for those a year old; and trains, stuffed animals, and toy cars were available for the toddlers. This playroom teacher (or "toy lady") introduced soon-to-be mobile children to the playroom.

At the beginning of their hospitalizations, many of the children were reluctant to venture into the unknown territory of the playroom. For this reason, a teacher was assigned to each child. Their hospitalizations had separated them from their parents, so patients needed to feel an extra measure of security, and the relationships that developed between teachers and patients were found to be vital to the wellbeing of the children. In the playroom,

Enjoying the fresh air at the Jackson Building. Taken circa 1960.

children had their own special teachers to whom they could go for comfort.

The patients could spend the whole day in the playroom, with time out when necessary for therapy or medication. Parents were welcomed during visiting hours, and later, those involved in living-in arrangements could spend the day there. Lunch was served to all the children every day at a small round table in the playroom. After lunch, children went back to their beds for a nap but returned to the playroom in the afternoon. Dinner was served on the wards, and afterwards the playroom came to the patients. Evening volunteers read to the children or played with them before bedtime.

Pajamas are not the most comfortable play clothes, so there was a playroom uniform: T-shirts and blue denim overalls or jeans with name tags attached. The teachers wore bright-colored smocks. For the children, the time spent in the playroom provided a happy contrast to the often frightening or painful treatments their illnesses inflicted on them.

Although it was also a learning place for the professionals who gained knowledge about the special needs of hospitalized and ill children, for the patients the playroom was just that, an area in which children played as they wished in a happy atmosphere that helped them forget they were hospitalized. Doctors were not allowed to do any medical procedures while their patients were in the playroom; it was a safe space for the children. One wall near the playroom was covered with the autographs of former patients and drawings they had made. Every few years, when the writing covered the surface, the wall was painted and soon a new group of autographs and drawings appeared.

Mrs. Angoff and Dr. Tisza shared their playroom experiences with their colleagues in several papers describing in great detail the philosophy, programs, and clinical findings of the play program.[2] For the lay reader, these papers reflect the happy spirit of the place, and the case histories reveal the warm feelings these professionals had for their patients.

Ms. Geneva Katz, administrator of the Floating, in an *American Journal of Nursing* article entitled "The Happy Ship," described how the playroom transformed the necessary hospital routine into fun. She tells of a little girl above whose crib was posted the notice: "Nothing by Mouth." The child was able to leave her crib, and it seemed cruel to keep her in her bed just to make sure that she would not be fed. She was able to move about in the corridor and the playroom because the nurses made up a "sandwich-board" of two signs printed on cardboard that were pinned on her pajamas. As Ms. Katz described it, "she pranced off gleefully with the instructions, Nothing By Mouth, decorating her small person, front and back."[3]

In the same article, Ms. Katz summed up the general atmosphere around the playroom by relating an anecdote about an elderly physician who visited the Floating:

"As he turned into one of the corridors he saw a five year old lad running as fast as his legs would carry him, arms outstretched to an approaching doctor. Without a moment's hesitation, the doctor swept his young friend into the expected embrace, and there was an affectionate exchange of greetings. This completely spontaneous, typical incident brought tears to the eyes of the visiting doctor, who confessed that he had come into the hospital expecting to find the efficient, scientifically operated institution with the usual cold, impersonal atmosphere.

"The science was there. The medical procedures were performed. It was, first of all, a pediatric hospital, but as Ms. Katz pointed out, for this young patient, 'The necessary treatments and medications have been overshadowed by his interest and his joyful participation in a normal happy living experience.'

Over the years, the playroom expanded. A library with a part-time librarian was added adjacent to the playroom, and tutors were on call for those children who were in the hospital for a protracted stay. Birthdays were celebrated with parties, and by the end of the 1970s there were monthly visits by a representative of the New England Aquarium who brought a sea animal in a portable tank of seawater. A portrait painter arrived once a month to make pastel portraits of the children, and other entertainers made appearances. Today, the playroom, part of the Child Life Program, remains an important area in the new Floating Hospital building. It is located on the eighth floor and was under the direction of Virginia Finn, Mrs. Angoff's successor, until 2012.

GETTING AND KEEPING PARENTS INVOLVED

One of the Floating's most important and far-reaching innovations grew out of the tradition established during the first years on the barge *Clifford* when parents had been a part of patient care. This involvement in the daily life at the hospital fostered a feeling of trust, and it strengthened the bonds between the nurses and parents that were considered an important part of the treatment of the patients. In the Jackson Building, as on the boat, parents were a vital part of the program assisting the nurses in caring for their children.

Because they were so involved during the day, many parents were reluctant to leave their children and go home in the evening. By 1954, an informal sleeping arrangement had been set up for those who wanted to spend the night. The parents who "lived in" were increasingly involved with their children's care. After a night spent on a foldout cot in the playroom (or whatever space could be found), a parent would be there in the morning to greet and feed her child breakfast. Parents were also on hand when children woke up during the night. They could comfort the fearful, read familiar bedtime stories, and generally reassure a small child who was in an unfamiliar place surrounded by strangers.

The small kitchen on the third floor was available to parents who wanted to bake cookies or make special treats for their children, and a sense of community developed among families who came from many different parts of the city and state. Their differences disappeared with the common bond they forged through their children.

Family participation was popular among parents and soon was an accepted part of a child's hospital stay. Not all parents were able to spend so much time at the hospital, but an increasing number wanted to. However, parents were not permitted to eat their meals in the hospital. The nurses established this rule for the parents' benefit, as they realized that parents needed to have some relief from the constant attention their children demanded.

After a few years of this somewhat informal arrangement, a formal Family Participation Unit (FPU) was established at the Floating. It grew out of a three-year design study launched in 1962.[4] The investigators (Dr. Marshall Kreidberg, Ms. Katz, architect Herman Field, architectural designer Delbert Highland, and social anthropologist Donald A. Kennedy) examined the special needs of the patients, their parents, and the doctors, nurses, technicians, and others involved in the care of hospitalized children. In 1979, the new Floating Hospital would be built as part of the New England Medical Center, and the study was charged with finding the best possible plan for the care of children. This also involved developing basic ideas about the architectural design and took into account the mission of a pediatric teaching hospital. One of the conclusions of the study focused on the needs of parents. It stated that visiting hours for parents should be flexible and parents should be able to stay with their children overnight in double rooms designed for that purpose.

The FPU was formally opened as a demonstration project in 1963. It was the first such unit in the country. Dr. Kreidberg, then the acting pediatrician-in-chief, saw the new unit as a way to forge an interaction between young medical students and the parents of their patients.[5] At first, many doctors were more resistant to the new unit than were nurses, who were used to working with parents. Nurses enthusiastically welcomed the help of the mothers and appreciated the positive impact their presence had on their patients.

As the new unit formalized the participation of the parents, it increasingly placed responsibility for certain aspects of their child's care on them. No longer were they there simply to comfort the child. Now, under the supervision of the nurses, mothers and fathers gave their children medications, bathed them, and accompanied them to as many tests and treatments as possible. And overnight, from 5:00 p.m. to 8:00 a.m., the parents were completely in charge. They put their children to sleep, were there in the morning when they woke up, and provided a sense of safety for anxious youngsters. This not only made the children less apprehensive about the hospital experience, it gave the parents a better understanding of the nature of the child's illness and the treatments that were administered.

The FPU instituted a screening process that ruled out children with behavior problems, as well as mothers who had psychological difficulties related to the child and were unable to cope with responsibilities related to the FPU. At the outset, admissions to the FPU were limited to medical and surgical diagnostic cases and to children hospitalized for simple treatments or minor surgeries.[6] This was broadened over the years as the staff gained experience in family participation. The FPU also featured Family Centered Medical Rounds, which urged the families to participate in their child's medical care. The doctors and staff strove to make parents and families their partners and to stress that they were not at the hospital only to comfort their child. When the tradition of Family Centered Medical Rounds first began, it was unique to the Floating. Many other hospitals were quick to adopt this innovative practice.

Because the parents contributed substantially to the care of their children, room rates were reduced by five dollars when they were in residence on the FPU, and there was no charge for their beds or for the snacks that were provided for the patients.

Each of the original FPU spaces consisted of a single room with a crib and a studio couch on which the mother or father slept. The room was furnished with bureaus and desks and decorated with pictures. The four rooms shared some basic kitchen facilities such as a toaster and refrigerator, and snack foods were available. There was also a hot plate for making tea or coffee. The original four-bed unit was soon increased to nine. Later, the private rooms on the fifth floor were also used.

The newspapers gave a great deal of space to the opening of the innovative FPU. Dr. Harold Wolman, director of child psychiatry at the Floating, was quoted in the press as he explained the genesis of the unit: "We know that when a child is hurt, he will turn to his mother or father. Yet when a child is sick, we traditionally take the child away from his parents. Often they feel it's a kind of punishment, which of course they don't understand."[7]

Dr. Kreidberg added, "After all, mom is a pretty capable person when she's at home. Why should she leave off all responsibilities for her child at the front door? It seems to us she can be a very great help in the hospital, too."[8]

It was true that, in many ways, the Floating hadn't changed. Its patients were treated with the same compassion that had been its hallmark from the start. An underlying understanding of the importance of treating the whole child and not just the disease continued to be the guiding principle. The professional staff was keenly aware that sick children had special psychological and physical needs that had to be taken into account. They were not just "little adults," but a distinct category of patients demanding special attention. At the Floating, they received it. To a remarkable extent, the principles that guided the hospital ship's philosophy continued to shape the direction the Floating took as it expanded and developed into an important component of a modern twentieth-century hospital complex.

The founders of the Floating had understood that the healing of children and their continued good health was intrinsically connected to the overall health of the family, as well as the interaction between hospital staff and the parents of the patients. The education of mothers, a priority on board the hospital ship, continued at the new hospital. In the early days on Ash Street, the Floating offered classes for mothers in special rooms in the basement. Later, parent involvement took a different, less-structured form. Parents were welcome and encouraged to participate in the care of the patients. During the years following World War II, this aspect of care was expanded in ways the founders of the Floating could never have foreseen.

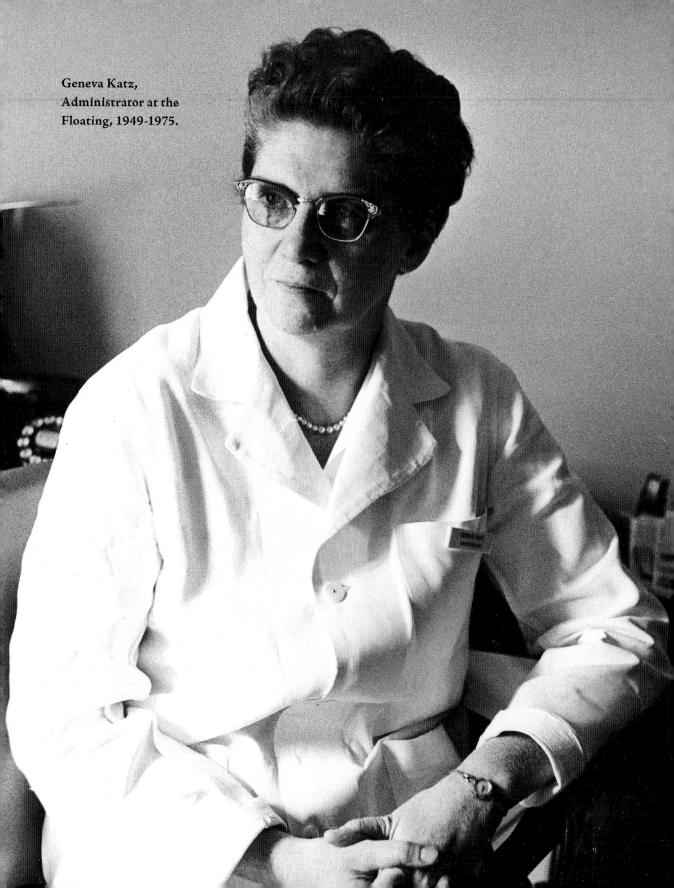

Geneva Katz,
Administrator at the
Floating, 1949-1975.

GENEVA KATZ

In 1949, Ms. Geneva Katz, R.N.[4] arrived at the Floating Hospital to assume the post of assistant administrator. Her vision of what a community pediatric hospital should be embodied many of the principles enunciated by the founders of the Floating Hospital. Her skillful direction of the hospital's program during the next decades resulted in changes in the care of sick children that had an impact on the many other pediatric hospitals that implemented her innovations.

Ms. Katz graduated from Ellis Hospital School of Nursing in Glens Falls, New York, in 1931 and took a job as an obstetrics nurse at the hospital. She worked six nights a week in twelve-hour shifts. After some time on this grueling schedule, she took a position in the operating room where the hours were better. She remained an operating room nurse for thirteen years, and by the beginning of World War II, she had been promoted to operating room supervisor.

In 1942, Ms. Katz tried to enlist in the Army Nurse Corps but was turned down for health reasons. She had spent more than a decade in nursing, and now her sights were set on enlarging her role in patient care with the goal of having an impact on her field. To achieve her objectives, she realized she would have to assume a position of authority and that meant going back to school.

With this goal in mind, Ms. Katz moved to Boston and enrolled at Boston University where she earned a degree in nursing education with a minor in business. After graduating in 1945, she signed a contract at Waltham Hospital as assistant administrator. She came to the Floating Hospital with three years of experience in hospital administration to her credit. Her twenty-six-year tenure at the Floating Hospital and the New England Medical Center coincided with a time of enormous change, growth, and development for the hospital, and for pediatrics and medicine as a whole. Her influence on the direction the Floating Hospital would take in the future was enormous.

When Ms. Katz arrived at the Floating Hospital, she was impressed by the hospital's innovative play program. Under the direction of Mrs. Kristine Angoff, a nursery school teacher with ten years of experience in the education of preschoolers, a lively nursery school was in full swing on the fourth floor from early in the morning until late in the afternoon. Designed to keep the patients happy and occupied, the playroom also gave the staff an opportunity to study how children responded to hospitalization.

In 1951, Ms. Katz became the administrator of the Floating Hospital. With new patients and an expanded service, the need to double the hospital's bed capacity seemed imperative. Ms. Katz transformed the storage space in the attic of the Jackson Building into a twenty-four-bed nursery connected by a ramp to the fourth floor nurse's dormitory. Twenty more beds were installed on the fourth floor of the Center Building. This added up to 101 beds, one more than the number the earlier survey had said was needed to make the Hospital economically viable. With the addition of the new beds, the hospital raised its fees to eleven dollars a day on the ward and thirteen dollars daily for a semiprivate room. By this time, health insurance payments began to help defray the cost of hospitalization and benefited the always-struggling hospital.

Ms. Katz's legacy can be seen at the Floating Hospital to this day. She worked with both patients and staff to fulfill her vision of what the hospital should be.

"The illustration shows the New England Medical Center building group as viewed from the southwest at the corner of Ash and Nassau Streets. At the right is the Center Building, which will be used jointly by the Tufts Medical School, the Boston Dispensary and the Boston Floating Hospital. On the corner stands the Floating Hospital's land hospital for babies and small children; while adjoining it, further to the left, are the Dispensary's present buildings, which will be remodeled and reorganized. The architects for the Center building were Andrews, Jones, Biscoe and Whitmore; for the Floating Hospital, Stevens and Lee, and for the Dispensary, Stickland, Blodget and Law; with Alfred Kellogg as consulting engineer." Architectural plans, date unknown.

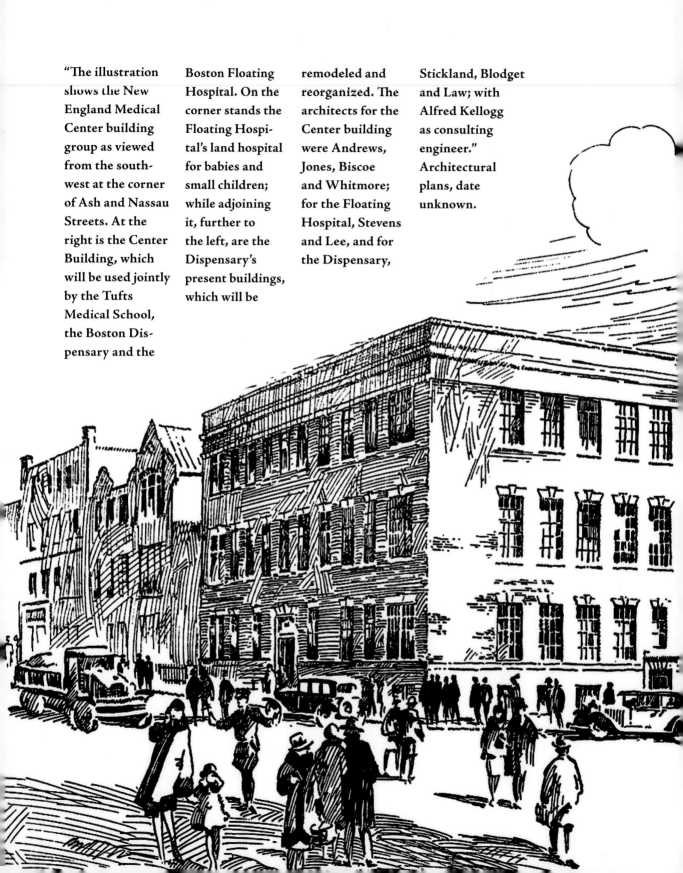

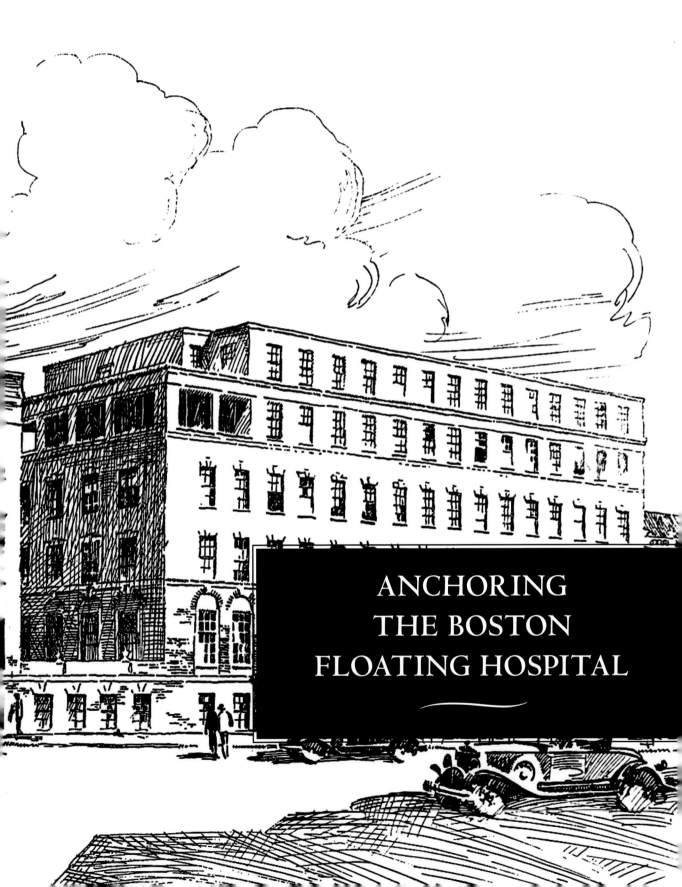

ANCHORING
THE BOSTON
FLOATING HOSPITAL

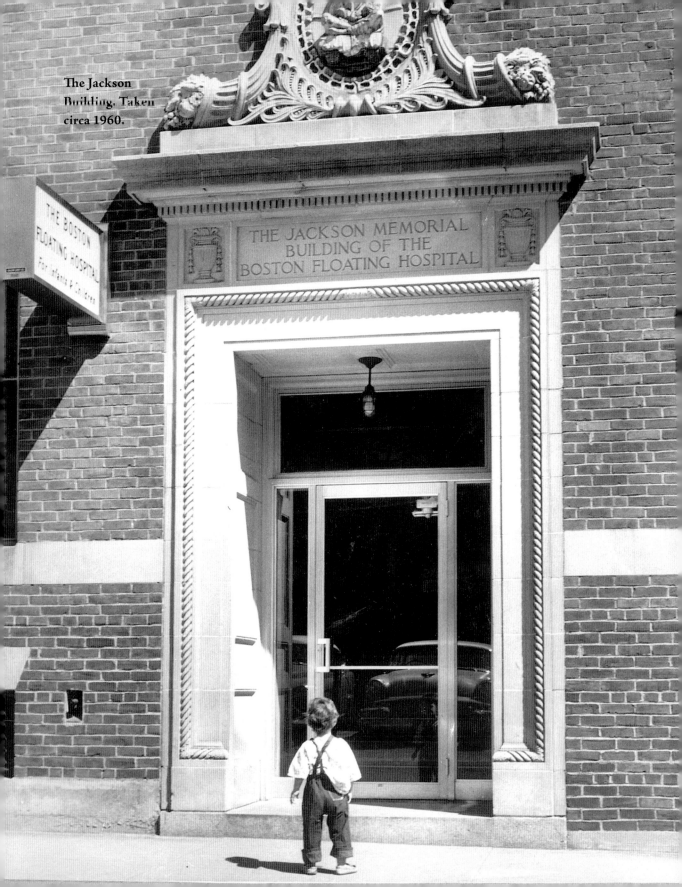

The Jackson Building, Taken circa 1960.

ANCHORING
THE BOSTON FLOATING HOSPITAL

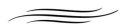

The growth and modernization of the Floating's facilities were placed on hold by the onset of World War II when, like all other hospitals in the country, it was beset by shortages of staff and difficulties in procuring supplies. Donations fell as support was shifted to the war effort, and necessary repairs and further expansion had to be deferred. But the war had an unexpected positive effect on the staff of the nearby Dispensary, which benefited from the influx of many distinguished refugee physicians from Germany and the occupied countries of Europe. Some of them also served at the Floating.

AFTER THE FIRE

The 1927 fire forced the Floating's board to take a hard look at the future of the institution. A committee of prominent doctors and philanthropists was appointed to study the changing needs of sick children in Boston. Like Lewis Freeman, they were aware that "conditions in child health had changed, partly as a result of the Floating's own research into the intestinal diseases of children and education about the need of better milk. The peak of childhood diseases no longer came in the summer." [1] At the same time, Mr. Freeman expressed a wistful nostalgia for the boat, which gave a bit of relief to "a tired mother with a helpless, sick or ailing infant tied to her home by her family's economic condition for whom little or no relief has been provided."

Those in charge of plotting the future of the Floating were less sentimental. On June 12, 1928, the physicians' committee published its report. It stated that, in their opinion, it was "inexpedient" to rebuild the boat. "Our conclusion is that the supplying of hospital service on a boat is not now the way in which the Floating can best carry out the purposes for which it was established." Edward W. Pope, president of The Boston Floating Hospital Corporation, listed one of the reasons for this decision: the board had estimated that the cost of one summer trip was equal to the cost of a whole year on land. [2]

While the board investigated ways of converting the Floating to a land-based institution, the Floating's patients would be seen at Boston Children's Hospital, Infants' Hospital, the Boston Dispensary, and the Children's Island Sanitarium off the coast of Marblehead. Doctors and nurses from the Floating would continue to supervise their care. The hospital's funds would be used for this purpose until new arrangements could be made.

Since its inception, the Floating had been closely allied with the Boston Dispensary; many of the doctors who served on the *Clifford* were from the Boston Dispensary. Because of their intertwined histories, the board of trustees favored the plan that would place the Floating's new building adjacent to the Boston Dispensary. An affiliation between the Boston Dispensary, the Floating, and Tufts Medical School was established in 1929, and in 1930, the Massachusetts Legislature authorized this entity, known as the New England Medical Center, to operate a medical center under the supervision of an administrative board composed of representatives from each institution. [3] The physician-in-chief of the Floating would become professor and chairman of the Department of Pediatrics at the Tufts Medical School. [4]

In 1930, Tufts and the two hospitals organized a joint fundraising campaign to support alterations to the Dispensary: construction of a new medical school and the Center Building, which would provide clinic expansion and space for service facilities for the three institutions. The Center Building was to be located in the vicinity of the Dispensary and new Jackson Building (Floating Hospital), which was already under construction.[5]

The architectural firm Stevens and Lee was selected to design the Jackson Building, and Canter Construction Co. was hired as the general contractor. Other builders were hired to erect the Center Building and refurbish the Dispensary. William Brainerd was called in to coordinate the very complicated project of erecting not only the Jackson Building but also the two other early components of the Medical Center. As a founding member of The Boston Floating Hospital Corporation, Mr. Brainerd was a direct link to the past. He had just opened his own architectural office in 1897 when the Floating's board purchased the barge *Clifford* and hired him to refurbish it. Mr. Brainerd served on the Floating's board of trustees as clerk for thirty years before retiring in 1927.

According to an unpublished memoir written by his son, Henry, Mr. Brainerd's job on the Medical Center project was not an easy one. He had to coordinate the work of three architects, two structural engineers, one mechanical engineer, one general contractor, and numerous sub-contractors. But Brainerd seems to have been up to the task. He was a meticulous and frugal man who once refused to pay a contractor's bill for rubber boots, asserting that it was the contractor's responsibility to outfit his workers. Not until the

Patients waiting outside the On-Shore Department on Wigglesworth Street. Taken in 1923.

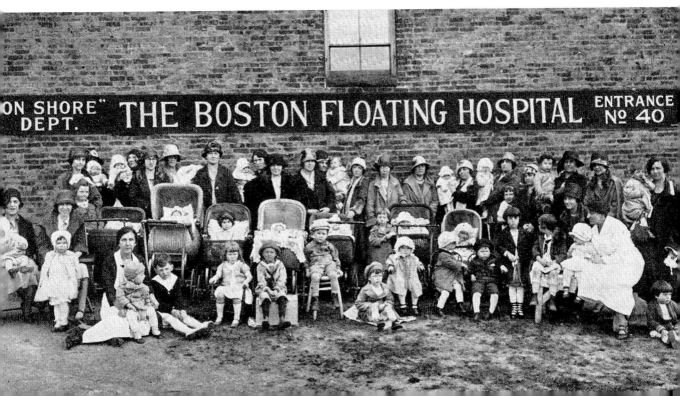

ON SHORE" DEPT. THE BOSTON FLOATING HOSPITAL ENTRANCE Nº 40

contractor explained that the boots would be practically destroyed from the heavy wear they would endure and would have to be discarded after the job was done did Mr. Brainerd approve the expenditure. [6]

ASH STREET

On October 12, 1931, the Floating opened its doors in the new Jackson Memorial Building at 20 Ash Street and began to admit patients. A report made to the Council on Medical Education of the American Medical Association by Dr. F.H. Arestad describes the physical plant of the new hospital: [7]

> "(It is a) four-story brick structure ... the first floor contains the admissions office with two examining rooms and a laboratory section, administrative offices, staff room and a space for the medical library. The second and third floors are used for patients accommodated in small wards having the cubicle arrangement. Each of these floors has a surgical dressing room, special diet kitchens, and facilities for isolation. A premature room is also available.
>
> "The fourth floor contains a sun room enclosed with Vitaglass, an open solarium, a play room, and a section which can be equipped with additional beds. In the basement there is a well-equipped lecture room used by the nurses training program. [8] Good autopsy facilities are also furnished in the basement.
>
> "In general it can be stated that the equipment and facilities are excellent for the special work which this hospital is undertaking ... it is evident that the entire staff consists of physicians who are specialists in the various fields of medicine and surgery and who are intimately connected with teaching in medical schools. The hospital is well equipped and staffed for the training of resident physicians in the specialty of pediatrics."

In fact, the Floating's new quarters quickly proved to be cramped, and the hospital was woefully underequipped. The Jackson Building had no operating rooms, no radiology unit, and diet kitchens so limited in size and scope that they could not serve all of the hospital's patients. There was only one elevator and one small linen closet. The only public bathroom was on the fourth floor, and there was no lounge area for staff or families of patients.

After the first full year in the Jackson Building, and despite its obvious physical shortcomings, the trustees of The Boston Floating Hospital concluded that the mandate under which the hospital had always operated—the care of the sick children of the poor, the study of childhood diseases, and the training of medical students and nurses as well as the provision of instruction to mothers—was being better fulfilled in the fifty-bed, year-round free hospital on land than on a boat that was operational only during the summer months.[9]

Until 1982, when it was moved into its current building, the hospital—like the other institutions in the medical center—bought the services it lacked from the Boston Dispensary. In time, the staff found ways to overcome the hospital's shortcomings, but there was no getting around the fact that the new Floating Hospital's patient capacity of forty beds was far smaller than it had been on board the boat.

These were hard times, and the size of the Floating and the number of its amenities were limited by the availability of funds. In spite of this, the hospital's staff was dedicated to continuing the Floating's tradition of delivering the very best care to the poor children of Boston. The children's inpatient ward of the Boston Dispensary was moved into the new Jackson Building, and one year after the new hospital opened, ten beds were added for a total of fifty.

In 1931, the Boston Dispensary opened a new twenty-bed diagnostic ward and clinic. By 1936, the diagnostic clinic was serving eight hundred patients annually. The William Bingham Association, which had long been supportive of the Boston Dispensary, provided the money to purchase the Franciscan Monastery of St. Clare, at the corner of Harrison Avenue and Bennet Street, in order to build a hospital on the site. The new hospital, named for Dr. Joseph Pratt, the Boston Dispensary's legendary chief-of-staff, was opened on December 15, 1938.

In a short time, the six-floor, one-hundred-bed Pratt Diagnostic Clinic (which continued to be known as the New England Center Hospital) became the largest diagnostic hospital in the nation. The Pratt's physician-in-chief, Dr. Samuel Proger, had arrived at the Boston Dispensary in 1929 as a medical student. Dr. Proger became a driving force in the establishment of the New England Medical Center (NEMC). On March 1, 1965, the Massachusetts Legislature approved the merger of all of the previously affiliated entities, excluding the medical school, into the New England Medical Center Hospitals (in 2008, the name was changed to Tufts Medical Center).

Until 1938, the Floating had always served all its patients without cost. That year, it began to charge five dollars a day in a newly set up semi-private ward of four beds. Three years later, fee-paying patients were admitted to the general wards. However, no child was ever turned away from the hospital because his or her parents were unable to pay.

After the 1927 fire and before the construction of the Jackson Building was completed in 1931, the Floating still managed to "sail" around the city of Boston in search of a permanent home. The ever-expanding hospital changed buildings several times before dropping anchor on Washington Street.

WASHINGTON STREET

By the 1960s, the Jackson Building was showing its age. Cracks opened up in the walls, the floors were worn, and there was a shabby look to the place. Repairs were made but often couldn't keep up with the wear and tear. But if parents—especially those who were well-to-do—were taken aback by their first look at the hospital, they quickly forgot the physical defects once they understood that their children were in a unique place where the priorities were not fancy decoration but first-rate medical care.

Ground was broken on the new Floating buildings in 1979. Taken in 1981.

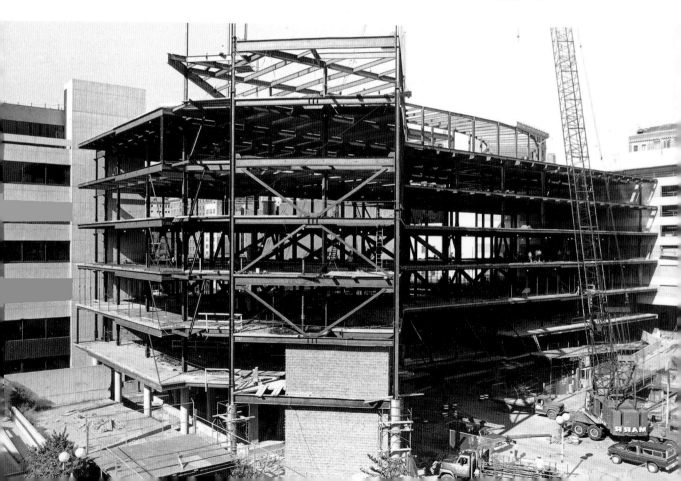

In 1974, after the Proger Building and the Tufts University School of Dental Medicine opened, it looked like the new Floating Hospital would finally be built. But when the NEMC applied for the required "certificate of need" from the State Public Health Council, the project, which was estimated to cost $51 million, was rejected as being too costly. It was not until late in 1977 that a new, less-expensive project was approved. Ironically, by the time of the building's groundbreaking ceremony in 1979, the estimated thirty-eight-million-dollar cost for construction had risen to fifty-five million dollars because of inflation. Most of the funds for building the Floating came through a Federal Housing Administration mortgage and a bond issue, and additional money was raised through a drive for funds launched in 1980 targeting private and public contributors.

A one-hundred-foot "bridge" of glass and steel, thirty-five feet above ground, connects the two parts of the building. Just one short flight above the lobby, a children's waiting room has been built in the shape of a boat. Miniature portholes can be seen from the street through the glass walls of the building. Inside the room, children can play in the "wheelhouse" and pretend they are sailing in the harbor. Today, most of them probably do not realize that the room was built as a fond tribute to an old hospital ship.

It seems fitting that the new Floating was built over the air rights on Washington Street, rising eight stories in a structure that seems to float above the street. The firm of Perry, Dean, Stahl and Rogers, specialists in hospital design, paid homage to the hospital's antecedents and were keenly aware that, although the hospital would have several other functions, it was primarily a hospital for children. Elizabeth Ericson, the project architect, told the *Boston Sunday Globe* that the new building aimed to "create a lively livable space, a kind of family room for the Center and the Community, full of activity and color. It is really designed as a big playground with ramps and lots of glass at ground level."[10]

Almost a century after the launching of the first hospital boat, the new 280,000-square-foot structure housed wards with ninety-six pediatric beds, four family participation rooms, twelve operating rooms for both adult and pediatric patients, a large playroom on the top floor, radiology departments for both adults and children, the laboratories for the entire medical center, and a pharmacy and pediatric walk-in clinic on the street level. Administrative and physician offices and clinic space for all subspecialties were housed throughout the new building.

A new tenant in the building was the Kiwanis Pediatric Trauma Institute, a joint program with Tufts Medical Center and the Floating that was the first of its kind in the country. The Kiwanis Foundation of New England, Tufts Medical Center, and other for profit and non-profit organizations sponsor this pediatric trauma unit. Hospitals from all over the region send children to the Floating's trauma center and the doctors who were trained to deal with unique pediatric injuries. The trauma center participates in the research and teaching program at the hospital, as well as in pediatric injury prevention education and outreach programs in the community.

In early July 1982, in a scene reminiscent of the 1906 transfer of patients from the old barge *Clifford* to the new Floating Hospital, patients were brought from 20 Ash Street to the new building by nurses and doctors.

Although the Floating contained fewer than the one hundred pediatric beds once thought necessary for a hospital's financial health, Dr. Sydney Gellis, pediatrician-in-chief, stated in a 1982 interview that these beds were for severely ill or injured patients and for children who lived in the Floating's neighborhood. Dr. Gellis said he "was not particularly concerned about bed numbers so long as large clinic areas were provided because children with defects that might have resulted in their deaths in the past are now living normal lives but require periodic outpatient follow-up by specialists. The beds are for the initial treatment of children who need special care."[11] Today, the hospital's outpatient facilities work at full capacity year-round.

LEADING AND EXPANDING
THE BOSTON FLOATING HOSPITAL

During the 1950s and 1960s, the Floating was a community-based hospital, relying heavily on physician referrals, where private doctors treated their own patients. The "full-time" staff consisted of one-and-a-half doctors; Dr. James Baty was the part-time chief and Dr. Marshall Kreidberg was the full-time pediatrician. Gradually, the Floating realized the need for specialists, and neurology, psychiatry, hematology, and cardiology divisions were established and staffed.

There was no labor and delivery service at the New England Medical Center until 1992 when one opened in the Proger Building. Neonatologists cared for newborns at St. Margaret's Hospital in Dorchester. When the new Boston Floating Hospital opened in 1982, it included space for a small neonatal intensive care unit and a special care nursery on the sixth floor. These services later moved to the new North Building.

Over time, many individuals made major contributions to the development of the Floating Hospital, but in the second half of the twentieth century, Dr. Gellis was preeminent in establishing it as a major pediatric research and teaching hospital in the area. He came to the Floating as pediatrician-in-chief in 1965 after serving as professor and chairman of pediatrics and acting dean at Boston University School of Medicine. Before he signed his contract, he had received a guarantee that a new pediatric hospital would be built and that the Boston Floating would not be swallowed up once the NEMC erected a complex of new buildings. It would take almost two decades before the promise was kept. Until then, Dr. Gellis had a small office in the Jackson Building.

With the arrival of Dr. Gellis, an internationally respected pediatrician, a full-time department of pediatrics was established. Under his leadership, research programs were developed that focused on the value of growth hormone for children with hypopituitarism, seizure control, the link between birth defects and chromosomal abnormalities, hepatitis, autism, and jaundice of the newborn. Divisions of infectious diseases and urology were added, and adolescent and intensive care services were developed. Educating medical students, residents, and practicing pediatricians was Dr. Gellis' most lasting

Dr. Kreidberg and Ms. Katz in the Jackson Building's old playroom. Date unkown.

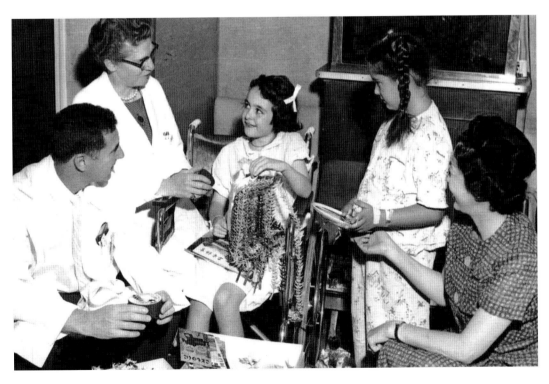

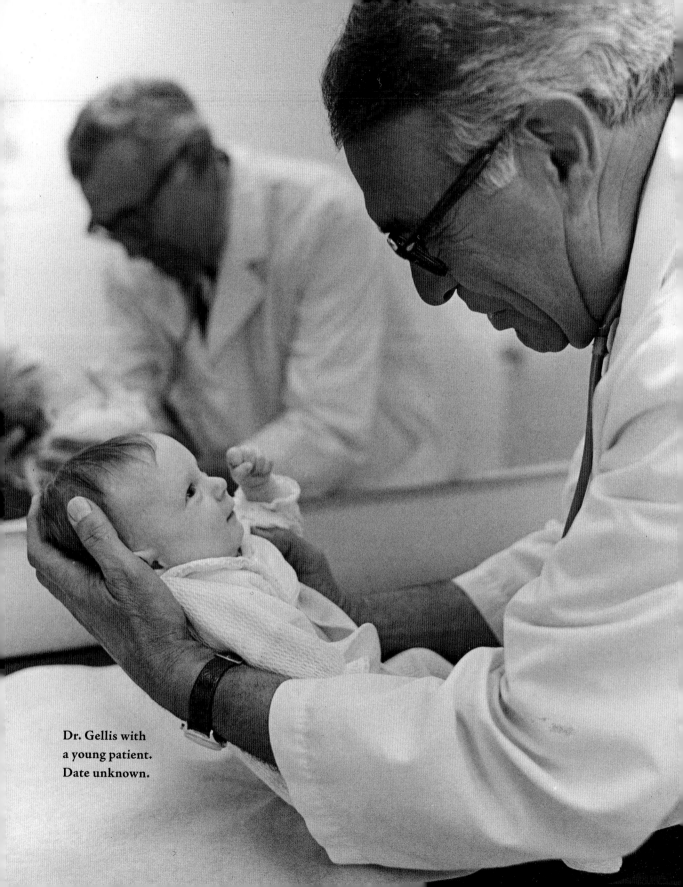

Dr. Gellis with
a young patient.
Date unknown.

legacy. The Floating was now firmly established as one of the most important pediatric research and teaching hospitals in the area. More than half of all the pediatricians who were practicing in New England in 1982 were trained at the Floating.[12] Dr. Gellis published a weekly *Pediatric Notes* newsletter that had a wide distribution to pediatricians all over the United States. The American Academy of Pediatrics honored his contributions to teaching on a national level by naming him a Pediatrics Pioneer in 1996.

Among the innovations Dr. Gellis instituted at the Floating was the Birth Defect Center sponsored by the March of Dimes Birth Defects Foundation. Later, the Tufts-New England Medical Center Birth Defects Information Service was established. This clearinghouse made it possible for hospitals around the country to receive and share information about birth defects.

In 1980, Dr. Gellis retired and was succeeded by Dr. Richard C. Talamo, an immunologist and professor of pediatrics at Johns Hopkins University School of Medicine. Dr. Talamo became seriously ill and died shortly after his appointment, and Dr. Kreidberg, a cardiologist, was named acting chief in 1981. Some of his innovations included the creation of an intensive care unit and a division of gastroenterology and nutrition.

Dr. Kreidberg served until Dr. Jane G. Schaller, an internationally recognized pediatric rheumatologist and children's rights advocate, became the Floating's pediatrician-in-chief and Leona and David Karp Professor of Pediatrics at the Tufts University School of Medicine in 1983. She had previously served as chief of the pediatric rheumatology service and professor of pediatrics at the University of Washington in Seattle.

Dr. Schaller tripled the physician staff and led the accreditation of nephrology and rheumatology divisions as well as fellowship-training programs in gastroenterology, neonatology, rheumatology, and adolescent medicine.

Mr. Freeman and Reverend Tobey would approve of the vision of today's Floating Hospital. In its outreach projects, the playroom, its Family Participation Unit, its research into the causes and cures of childhood diseases, and its emphasis on answering the need for good medical care in the community, the Floating Hospital of today, like the boat in 1894, uses all the resources at its disposal to fulfill the aims stated in 1895 by its founders in the first annual report: "The Floating Hospital is designed first of all for sick babies, everything else giving way to the plan and purpose to do all that possibly can be done to start the baby on the road to health."

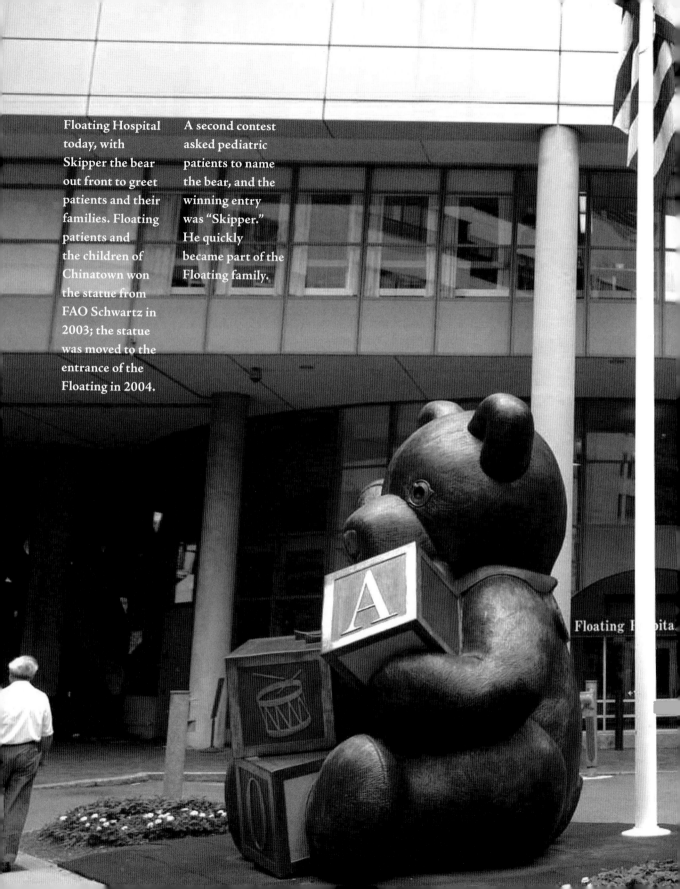

Floating Hospital today, with Skipper the bear out front to greet patients and their families. Floating patients and the children of Chinatown won the statue from FAO Schwartz in 2003; the statue was moved to the entrance of the Floating in 2004.

A second contest asked pediatric patients to name the bear, and the winning entry was "Skipper." He quickly became part of the Floating family.

POST SCRIPT

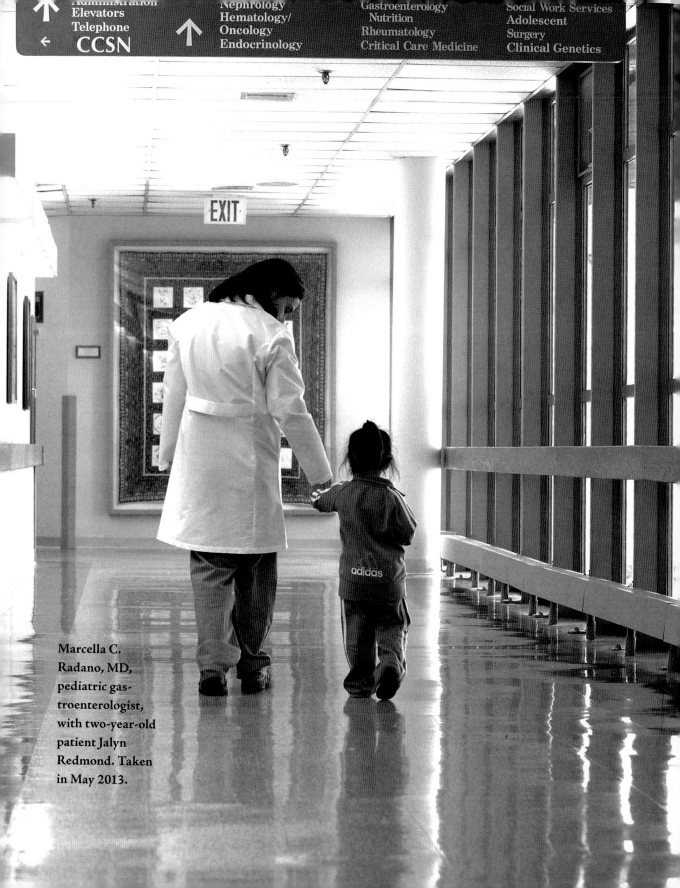

Administration
Elevators
Telephone
← CCSN

Nephrology
Hematology/
Oncology
Endocrinology

Gastroenterology
Nutrition
Rheumatology
Critical Care Medicine

Social Work Services
Adolescent
Surgery
Clinical Genetics

EXIT

adidas

Marcella C.
Radano, MD,
pediatric gas-
troenterologist,
with two-year-old
patient Jalyn
Redmond. Taken
in May 2013.

POST SCRIPT

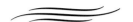

Since this history was written in the early 1990s, much has changed in the practice of medicine in the United States. In an effort to adapt to ever-changing regulatory mandates and fiscal constraints, hospitals have often merged in an effort to consolidate their clinical, research, and academic resources. The Floating continues to adapt and innovate in order to fulfill its mission to provide excellent, affordable, and family-centered care during these turbulent times.

Dr. Jane Schaller retired from the chairmanship and was succeeded in 1997 by Dr. Ivan D. Frantz, III, who came to the Floating from Boston Children's Hospital in 1985 as chief of newborn medicine. He developed an extensive network of Level 2 and Special Care Nurseries at community hospitals north and south of Boston. Dr. John R. Schreiber succeeded Dr. Frantz in 2007.

Dr. Schreiber, an infectious diseases specialist, was interested in vaccine development, particularly in increasing the immunogenicity and reducing the number of doses of conjugate vaccines such as pneumococcal. Before coming to the Floating, he had been the Ruben-Bentson Chair and Professor of Pediatrics and the head of the Department of Pediatrics at the University of Minnesota Medical School. Dr. Schreiber successfully focused on expanding the patient base and the Floating's local and national reputation.

Under his leadership, the Floating expanded to become the first integrated system for pediatric care in Boston. Through an extensive network, the Floating could maintain care management of many less-complex inpatient cases in the community through its on-site pediatric hospitalists and neonatologists. The growing number of patients meant the hospital could reinvest in its faculty; the Floating welcomed fifty-five new faculty members from 2007 to 2013. Research, presentations at national meetings, and residency applications all achieved new levels due to this growth.

The Floating's pediatric residency program dates back to 1932, just after the hospital came on shore. It has grown and flourished ever since and is especially appreciated for its intimate size. Residents gain a depth and breadth of clinical experience through exposure to the ethnically diverse populations they see at community hospitals, in the downtown location, and through close faculty relationships and strong mentorships. Individualized education that focuses on each resident's career plans is available via three tracks that address: (1) care of the acutely ill child; (2) primary care and development; and (3) pediatric subspecialty care. Quality of care and patient safety were and are integral components of training.

Since its earliest days, research has been a part of the Floating's mission. Faculty members have received significant National Institutes of Health (NIH) and NIH-equivalent funded grants. There are four principal areas of research that investigators have been exploring in the last twenty years: (1) developmental and behavioral disorders, such as autism, learning disabilities, attention deficit hyperactivity disorder (ADHD), and cerebral palsy; (2) neonatal investigations into lung biology and lung development, perinatal epidemiology, prevention of preterm birth and its complications, and biomechanics of the cervix; (3) genetic, genomic, and proteomic approaches to the diagnosis and treatment of various perinatal and pediatric problems; and (4) pediatric precursors of adult disease to examine how maternal health issues during pregnancy, such as obesity and diabetes, affect child health, from a cardiovascular, metabolic, and behavioral perspective.

Maintaining and modernizing the physical plant and equipment at the Floating has also received ongoing attention. In recent years, hospital administrators have added a new bone marrow transplant unit, a pediatric catheterization lab, an outpatient oncology clinic, a conscious sedation unit, and completed inpatient ward renovations, with many more renovations and upgrades planned for the near future.

The accomplishments of the hospital and its staff have far exceeded the modest goals Reverend Tobey established for The Boston Floating Hospital with his supporters 120 years ago. As Dr. Sydney Gellis wrote in a *Tufts Medical Alumni Bulletin* in 1966, "The Boston Floating Hospital, despite the many advances in all areas of pediatrics, will maintain as its constant goal the interest and concern with the total child within his family and community setting." [1]

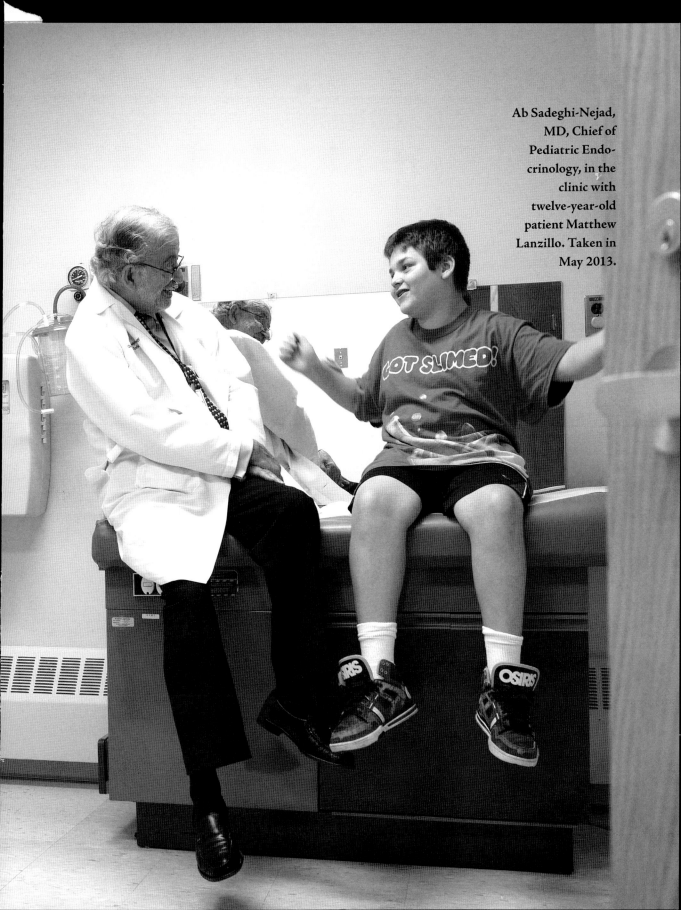

Ab Sadeghi-Nejad, MD, Chief of Pediatric Endocrinology, in the clinic with twelve-year-old patient Matthew Lanzillo. Taken in May 2013.

BOSTON FLOATING HOSPITAL
CHIEFS OF SERVICE

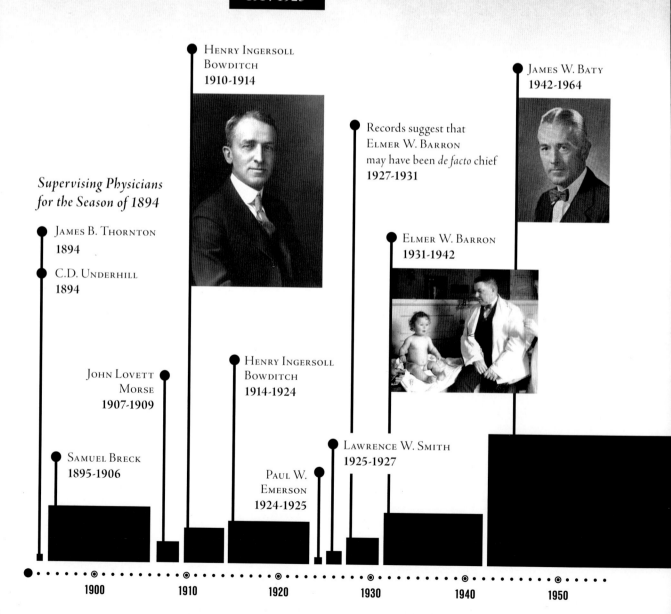

Chairs of Visiting Staff 1895-1913

Physician-In-Charge 1914-1925

Chief of Staff 1914-1964

HENRY INGERSOLL BOWDITCH
1910-1914

JAMES W. BATY
1942-1964

Records suggest that
ELMER W. BARRON
may have been *de facto* chief
1927-1931

Supervising Physicians for the Season of 1894

JAMES B. THORNTON
1894

C.D. UNDERHILL
1894

ELMER W. BARRON
1931-1942

JOHN LOVETT MORSE
1907-1909

HENRY INGERSOLL BOWDITCH
1914-1924

SAMUEL BRECK
1895-1906

LAWRENCE W. SMITH
1925-1927

PAUL W. EMERSON
1924-1925

1900   1910   1920   1930   1940   1950

Pediatrician-In-Chief 1965-2013

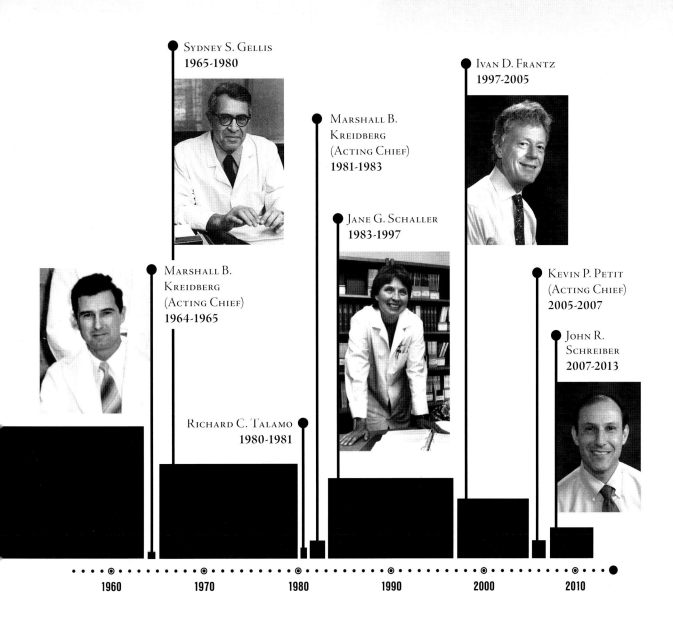

SYDNEY S. GELLIS
1965-1980

MARSHALL B. KREIDBERG (ACTING CHIEF)
1981-1983

IVAN D. FRANTZ
1997-2005

MARSHALL B. KREIDBERG (ACTING CHIEF)
1964-1965

JANE G. SCHALLER
1983-1997

KEVIN P. PETIT (ACTING CHIEF)
2005-2007

JOHN R. SCHREIBER
2007-2013

RICHARD C. TALAMO
1980-1981

1960   1970   1980   1990   2000   2010

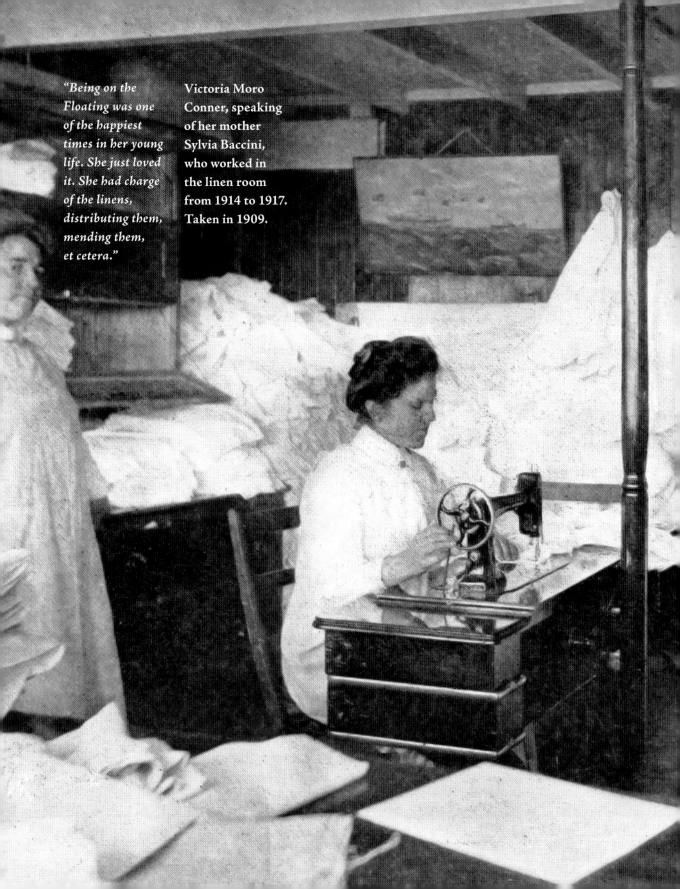

"Being on the Floating was one of the happiest times in her young life. She just loved it. She had charge of the linens, distributing them, mending them, et cetera."

Victoria Moro Conner, speaking of her mother Sylvia Baccini, who worked in the linen room from 1914 to 1917. Taken in 1909.

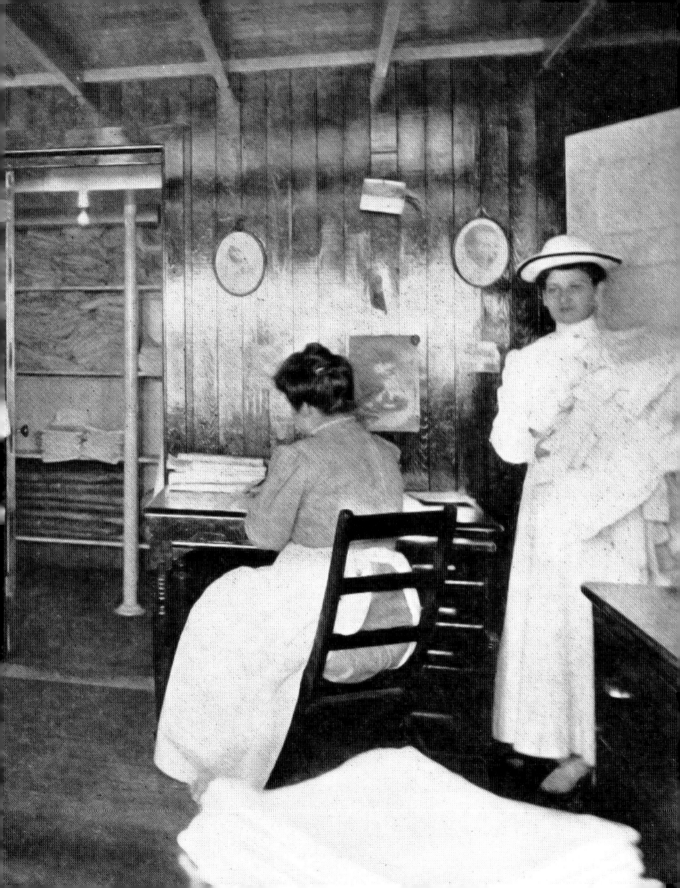

ACKNOWLEDGEMENTS

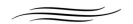

In the early 1990s Dr. Jane Schaller, then Chairman of Pediatrics at Tufts Medical Center, asked me to write a history of the Floating Hospital as its 100th anniversary approached. Prior to my involvement, Dr. Schaller's medical editor, Mary Sullivan had interviewed many of the ship's former staff, patients and parents. She had also done a significant amount of research on the social, economic and scientific trends of the mid 1800s to the early 1900s. Her well documented research was invaluable to me, as it provided context and background on the era. Dr. John Bowers' short unpublished history of the Floating also provided interesting details about the first two years on the *Clifford*. Drs. Sydney Gellis and Marshall Kreidberg, and Geneva Katz gave me firsthand accounts of the administrative and clinical development of the hospital during the 1950s and 60s and Christine Angoff and Virginia Finn invited me to observe their management of the Playroom. Dr. John Kulig, Director of Adolescent Medicine at the Floating, researched and presented Pediatric Grand Rounds on the history of the Floating and took the initiative to get this manuscript published after a twenty-year hiatus. He contributed to the book's chapter on the nurses and the critical role they played on the ship and on shore; played a key role in shaping and finalizing the manuscript; and worked closely with the publishers to ensure accuracy. Dr. Richard Grand, former Chief of Pediatric Gastroenterology/Nutrition at the Floating, also made insightful suggestions on substance and style.

Elizabeth Richardson and her colleagues at the Hirsh Health Sciences Library at Tufts University School of Medicine were of tremendous assistance in locating references and developing the bibliographic notes for the manuscript. Susanne Belovari of the Digital Collections and Archives at the Tisch Library at Tufts University in Medford made photos and newspaper clippings of the early days of the ship available to the book's editorial team.

Dan Bird, chairman of the Tufts Medical Center's Legacy Committee was instrumental in collecting the dispersed archives and arranging for their safe keeping at Tufts University. He also joined in the planning, discussion and reading through the chapters, offering his unique perspective throughout the process.

An enormous thank you goes to Jacoba van Schaik, who until 2011 was the academic affairs manager in the Department of Pediatrics. Her tireless efforts have driven the book to completion. Her detailed review of the hospital's annual reports and other relevant literatuare, her management of the original sources and footnotes, her input and endless rereads of the chapters, and the time she spent discovering and selecting the photographs were vital to this project. This book would have never come to be published without her.

I would also like to thank Deepa Chungi and Nicole Vecchiotti of Union Park Press for their strong commitment and editorial support. Their efforts, coupled with the dedication of Dr. Kulig, Mr. Bird, and Ms. van Schaik ensured that this history was published in recognition of the 120th anniversary of the launching of the Boston Floating Hospital.

Lucie Prinz

ENDNOTES

PROLOGUE

1. Samuel Rezneck, "Unemployment, Unrest, and Relief in the United States during the Depression of 1893-97," *Journal of Political Economy* 6, 4 (August 1953), 324-327.

2. Bureau of Statistics and Labor, Massachusetts, "24th Annual Report of the Bureau of Statistics of Labor. Current Statistical Matter Relating to Local Conditions: Unemployment in Massachusetts" (Boston, 1894), 114-240.

VICTORIAN BOSTON

1. Charles Dickens, *American Notes for General Circulation* (London: Chapman & Hall, 1850), 42.

2. "Total population, by sex and age: 1850–1990" (Table Aa185-286) and "Population of cities with at least 100,000 population in 1990: 1790–1990" (Table Aa832-1033) in *Historical Statistics of the United States* (Millennial edition online), Susan B. Carter et al., eds. (New York: Cambridge University Press, 2006).

3. "Infant Mortality," Seventh Report of the Massachusetts Board of Health, 496, in Albert H. Busk, *A Treatise on Hygiene and Public Health* (New York: William Wood, 1879), 272.

4. Lemuel Shattuck, *Report to the Committee of the City Council Appointed to Obtain the Census of Boston for the year 1845* (Boston: City Printer, 1846), 157.

5. Charles E. Rosenberg, *The Care of Strangers, The Rise of America's Hospital System* (New York: Basic Books, 1987), 4.

6. Ibid., 122.

7. Ibid., 17.

8. Children's Hospital, "Third Annual Report, 1871," 7-8, quoted in Morris J. Vogel, *The Invention of the Modern Hospital, Boston, 1870-1930* (Chicago: University of Chicago Press, 1980), 24.

9. Ibid.

10. F.M. Crandall, "The Modern Child," editorial in *Archives of Pediatrics* 15 (1898), 280.

11. Shattuck, *Report to the Committee*, 157.

12. Lemuel Shattuck, "The Vital Statistics of Boston, Containing an Abstract of the Bills of Mortality for the Last Twenty-Nine Years and a General View of the Population and Health of the City at Other Periods of its History," *American Journal of the Medical Sciences* 1 (1841), 369-400.

13. Thomas E. Cone, *History of American Pediatrics* (Boston: Little Brown, 1979), 76.

14. Ibid., 105.

15. Ibid., 104.

16. Ibid., 102-103.

FOUNDING EFFORTS: RAISING MONEY AND FULFILLING THE MANDATE

1. Chronological information about the voyages of the Floating Hospital ship, statistics, staff, and funds come from Boston Floating Hospital Annual Reports [BFH], 1894-1927, in Digital Collection & Archives [DCA], Tufts University,

Medford, Massachusetts. All other unpublished materials cited are held at DCA.

2. Lewis A. Freeman, "The Boston Floating Hospital," March 1933, 2-4.

3. "Lewis Freeman on Leave of Absence from the Boston Floating Hospital," interview by Elsie Briggs, Greenwood, Massachusetts, March 1933, 1-4.

Early Fundraising Efforts

4. BFH, *History, Season of 1898*, 4.

5. Harriet Osgood, "The Babies' Outing: A Day on the Floating Hospital and its Second Trip Down the Harbor," *Boston Sunday Post*, July 21, 1895.

6. Edward E. Hale, *Boston Floating Hospital*, 1898, 8.

7. "Will Labor in New Field," *Boston Herald*, November 9, 1895.

8. Boston's Infants' Hospital started as the West End Nursery in 1881 on Blossom Street. By 1884 it was known as the West End Nursery and Infants' Hospital. In 1902 the name was changed to The Thomas Morgan Rotch Jr. Memorial Hospital, but in 1907 it was changed back to Infants' Hospital. In 1914 the hospital moved to Shattuck Street, and in 1923 it moved again to land acquired by Children's Hospital. In 1961 it merged with Children's Hospital. Both the nursery and Boston's Infants' Hospital were designed to care for infants and children under two years of age, who were too young to be treated at Children's Hospital.

9. "CHARITY MONEY: How Many Thousands Have Gone into Shrewd Speculators' Pockets," *Boston Post*, November 11, 1895.

10. BFH, *Season of 1895*, 6.

An Experimental Success! New Needs Arise

11. "A Hundred Happy Babies: Sick Children Taken Down to Harbor on the First Trip of This Year of the Boston Floating Hospital," *Boston Transcript*, July 11, 1896.

12. Osgood, "The Babies' Outing."

13. "Coaxed Back to Roses: Little Children Gain Color on Floating Hospital," *Boston Globe*, July 24, 1895.

Changing Attitudes Towards Poor Mothers

14. BFH, *History and Report, Season of 1900*, 37.

15. BFH, *Season of 1894*, 5.

16. BFH, *Season of 1900*, 33.

17. The Boston Floating Hospital, *Home Directions for Mother to Sterilize Milk*, 1897.

TURN OF THE CENTURY: A NEW ERA FOR THE FLOATING HOSPITAL

Buying the New Ship

1. BFH, *Twelfth Annual Report, Season of 1905*, 9-10.

2. BFH, *Report, Season of 1904*, 16.

Raising Funds for the New Boat

3. BFH, *Season of 1905*, 4.

4. BFH, *Report, Season of 1901*, 5.

5. BFH, *Report, Season of 1902*, 3-4.

6. The Boston Floating Hospital, *Historical Sketch* (1903), 25.

7. BFH, *Season of 1904*, 5.

8. Ibid., 8.

Plans for the Ship

9. Ibid., 9.

10. BFH, *Season of 1905*, 10.

11. "The Boston Floating Hospital, A Day on the 'White Ship of Mercy," *The Nurse, Journal of Practical Knowledge* (January 1917), 10.

12. BFH, *Eighteenth Annual Report, Season of 1922*, 8.

1906 and the New Boat

13. Josephine Halberstadt, "The Boston Floating Hospital, Season of 1906," *American Journal of Nursing* 7, 4 (1907), 368-371.

14. BFH, *Thirteenth Annual Report, Season of 1906*, 7.

15. Ibid., 8.

16. Ibid., 19.

17. BFH, *Fourteenth Annual Report, Season of 1907*, 7.

MILK: THE PERFECT FOOD

Milk at the Floating Hospital

1. BFH, *Sixteenth Annual Report, Season of 1909*, 7.
2. R.M. Smith, "Two Types of Infectious Diarrhea"; A.I. Kendall, A.A. Day, "Observations on Summer Diarrheas in Children"; A.I. Kendall, "Observations on the Etiology of Severe Summer Diarrheas of Bacterial Causation," *Boston Medical and Surgical Journal*, CLXIX (November 20, 1913), 753-758.

3. BFH, *Season of 1909*, 8.

4. Oliver Wendell Holmes, "Scholastic and Bedside Teaching: Introductory Lecture to the Medical Class of Harvard University, Nov. 6, 1867," *Medical Essays 1842-1882* (Boston: Houghton Mifflin, 1883), 276.

5. Charles E. North, "Milk and its Relation to Public Health," in *A Half Century of Public Health*, ed. M.P. Ravenel (New York: American Public Health Association, 1921), 242.

Denny and Bosworth

6. BFH, *Twentieth Annual Report, Season of 1913*, 7.

7. "Mr. Bosworth," interview by David H. Brown, *Columbus (Ohio) Citizen*, 1965.

8. BFH, *Twenty-sixth Annual Report, Season of 1919*, 7.

9. Ibid., 8-9.

10. BFH, *Twenty-seventh and Twenty-eighth Annual Reports, Seasons of 1920 and 1921*, 7.

11. J. C. Runders, *The House That Similac Built* (Columbus, Ohio: Ross, 1968), 4-5.

12. Ibid., 5.

13. BFH *Twenty-ninth Annual Report, Season of 1922*, 5.

BACKGROUND ON MILK

Pasteurization

1. North, "Milk," 216-289.

2. Blondeau, "De la pré-existence et de l'invariabilités des germs," *Comptes Rendus Hebdomadaires des Séances de L'Académie des Sciences* (1847), 359-60.

3. "Pasteurization," *Encyclopedia Britannica*, online academic edition (2013).

4. North, "Milk," 270.

5. "Of the Inspection and Sale of Milk," *Massachusetts Public Statutes* Title X. Ch. 57 (1864-1880), 372-373.

6. E. Hart, "A Report on the Influence of Milk in Spreading Zymotic Disease," *The British Medical Journal* (May 5, 1897), 1231.

7. North, "Milk," 241.

8. Ibid., 267.

9. Ibid., 267-268.

Feeding Stations

10. Cone, *History*, 144.

11. Ibid.

12. North, "Milk," 279.

13. North, "Milk," 278.

14. "Clean Your Plate: Farming in Needham," Needham Historical Society, accessed March 2014, http://needhamhistory.org/features/articles/clean-your-plate.

15. Cone, *History*, 137.

16. North, "Milk," 278.

17. Ibid., 279.

18. BFH, *Seventeenth Annual Report, Season of 1910*, 12.

19. North, "Milk," 269.

20. Ibid., 241.

MEDICAL BREAKTHROUGHS AT THE FLOATING HOSPITAL

Evolution of the Food Lab

1. BFH, *Season of 1901*, 8.

2. BFH, *Season of 1902*, 18.

Sterilization and Pathology

3. Vogel, *The Invention*, 60-61.

4. BFH, *Season of 1901*, 13-19.

Air Conditioning and Air Quality

5. BFH, *Report, Season of 1899*, 7.

6. BFH, *Season of 1898*, 5-6.

7. BFH, *Season of 1900*, 30-31.

8. BFH, *Season of 1899*, 7-8.

Simon Flexner and Polio

9. BFH, *Annual Report, Season of 1903*, 7.

10. Ibid.

11. "Causes of Death Nosologically Arranged. Table X. I. l: Miasmatic" in *Annual Report on the Vital Statistics of Massachusetts: Births, Marriages, Divorces and Deaths* 52 (Boston: Commonwealth of Massachusetts Secretary of State, 1893), 56.

12. Benjamin Rush, "An Inquiry into the Causes and Cure of *Cholera Infantum*," in his *Medical Inquiries and Observations* 1 (Philadelphia: Thomas Dobson, 1794), 159-169.

13. Cone, *History*, 78-79.

14. Ibid., 79-80.

15. G.F. Powers, "Developments in Pediatrics in the Past Quarter Century," *Yale Journal of Biology and Medicine* 12:1 (1939-1940), 4.

16. George F. Still, *Common Disorders and Diseases of Childhood*, 2nd ed. (London: Henry Frowde, 1912), 211-231.

Medical Advances and Research

17. "A Day on the White Ship of Mercy," *The Nurse, Journal of Practical Knowledge* (January 1917), 4.

18. Ibid., 5-6.

19. BFH, *Season of 1913*, 9.

20. BFH, *Season of 1922*, 8-9; and BFH, *Thirty-first Annual Report, Season of 1924*, 9-10.

21. BFH. *Thirtieth Annual Report, Season of 1923*, 7.

X-Rays and Whooping Cough

22. BFH, *Season of 1923*, 8.

23. Ibid.

24. BFH, *Thirty-third Annual Report, Season of 1926*, 5.

25. Ibid., 8.

26. Ibid., 7.

Solarium

27. Lawrence Smith, *Report to Mr. Edward W. Pope, Chairman, Board of Trustees, Boston Floating Hospital*, March 23, 1925.

28. BFH, *Season of 1924*, 7.

29. Ibid.

Expanded Departments and Clinics

30. BFH, *Twenty-third Annual Report, Season of 1916*, 7.

31. BFH, *Season of 1926*, 9.

Polio

32. A.S. Pope, et al., "Evaluation of Poliomyelitis Vaccination in Massachusetts: From the Massachusetts Department of Public Health." *New England Journal of Medicine*, 254, 3 (January 19, 1956), 110-111.

Croup and Humidifiers

33. Geneva Katz, "A New Humidification Unit," n.d.

NURSES

1. BFH, *Season of 1901*, 7.

2. BFH, *Season of 1900*, 38.

3. R.W. Hastings, "The Boston Floating Hospital," *American Journal of Nursing* 6, 7 (April 1905), 436-437.

4. J.L. Henderson, "The Statistics of Prematurity: a Plea for Standardization," *Archives of Disease in Childhood* 21 (1946), 106.

CHANGING WITH THE TIMES

1. BFH, *Season of 1902*, 17.

2. BFH, *Season of 1900*, 19.

Changing Leadership

3. Ibid., 27.

4. Ibid.

5. "Death of Rev. Rufus R. Tobey," *Boston Evening Transcript*, January 6, 1920, 28.

6. Tobey obituary, *The Congregationalist*, January 1920.

7. Paul Beaven, ed., "History of the Boston Floating Hospital," *Pediatrics* 19, 4 (April 1957), 637.

On-Shore Department

8. BFH, *Eighteenth Annual Report, Season of 1911*, 7-8.

9. BFH, *Season of 1916*, 6.

10. "USN Ships – USS Boston Floating Hospital," U.S. Department of the Navy. Naval Historical Center ID #2366, accessed November 2012, http://www.history.navy.mil/photos/sh-usn/usnsh-b/id2366.htm.

11. BFH, *Thirtieth Annual Report, Season of 1923*, 5.

12. BFH, *Season of 1926*, 6.

Fire

13. "Floating Hospital is Destroyed by Fire," *Boston Globe*, June 2, 1927.

14. Filena Steward Robinson, interview by Mary Sullivan, June 13, 1989.

15. "USN Ships."

Major Contributors

16. Herbert Black, *Doctor and Teacher, Hospital Chief: Dr. Samuel Proger and the New England Medical Center* (Chester, Connecticut: Globe Pequot Press, 1982), 34.

After the Fire

17. "Lewis Freeman on Leave of Absence," 1933.

18. Black, *Doctor and Teacher*, 33.

19. Henry H. Banks, *A Century of Excellence, The*

History of Tufts University School of Medicine, 1893-1993 (Boston: Tufts University, 1993), 229.

20. Beaven, "History," 638.

21. Press release to Boston papers, New England Medical Center, January 26, 1931.

22. Henry Bowen Brainerd, "Memories of the Boston Floating Hospital," 1967, 5.

THE BOSTON FLOATING HOSPITAL AND FAMILIES
The Playroom

1. Rowland G. Freeman, "Playroom," *Report of the Psychiatric Service, Boston Floating Hospital*, 1951.

2. Veronica B. Tisza and Kristine Angoff, "A Play Program and its Function in a Pediatric Hospital," *Pediatrics* 19 (January 1957), 293-302; "A Play Program, the Role of the Playroom Teacher," *Pediatrics* 28 (November 1961), 841-5; and with Irving Hurwitz, "The Use of a Play Program by Hospitalized Children," *Journal of the American Academy of Child Psychiatry* 9 (July 1970), 515-31.

3. Geneva Katz, "The Happy Ship," *American Journal of Nursing* (May 1952).

Getting and Keeping Parents Involved

4. Geneva Katz, "Forty Years of Nursing," Graduation Address, Ellis Hospital School of Nursing, 1971, 8-11.

5. Loretta McLaughlin, "Mother Stays with Sick Child, Hospital Has Family Unit," *Boston Record American*, October 18, 1963.

6. Geneva Katz, "Mothers Help Take Care of Sick Children," *Hospitals, Journal of the American Hospital Association* 38 (July 1, 1964), 91.

7. Timothy Leland, "Mother is the Nurse, Home-in-Hospital Plan Started," *Boston Herald*, October 18, 1963.

8. Ibid.

ANCHORING THE FLOATING HOSPITAL
Ash Street

1. F.H. Arestad, "Report to the Council on Medical Education and Hospitals of the American Medical Association, July 15, 1932," in BFH, *Annual Report* (1932), 6.

2. The Floating Hospital conducted pediatric nurses training programs beginning on its first voyage in 1894. During the first few years, nurses were volunteers. At the turn of the century all nursing staff were graduates of nursing schools from as far away as Australia and were compensated. Housing for them was arranged at Maverick Square House in East Boston. Once the hospital became land-based, arrangements for trainee housing were made in nearby facilities; the Hemenway House on Nassau Street was a nurses' dormitory until 1970. In the course of time training programs were developed for both post-graduate and undergraduate nurses; some lasting six months, others two or three months. A 1952 *Handbook for Physicians and Parents* lists thirteen schools of nursing in Massachusetts, Maine, New Hampshire, and Vermont

that sent trainees for three months to the Floating's School of Affiliation in Pediatric Nursing. The training program ended in the early seventies.

3. Black, *Doctor and Teacher*, 33.

Washington Street

4. "A Major Hospital as a Kind of Family Room," *Boston Sunday Globe*, November 25, 1979.

5. Black, *Doctor and Teacher*, 166-167.

6. Ibid., 162.

POSTSCRIPT

1. Sydney S. Gellis, "The Boston Floating Hospital for Infants and Children," *Tufts Medical Alumni Bulletin*, March 1966, 9.

BOXES

1. BFH, *Annual Report* (1897), 12.

2. "A Philanthropist, B.C. Clark, Friend of Condemned Prisoners Generally," *Boston Advertiser*, May 7, 1897.

3. BFH, *Historical Sketch* (1903), 26-27.

4. Geneva Katz, interview by author, Boston Massachusetts, March 8, 1994.

INDEX

PHOTO CREDITS

Pages iv and v: The Boston Floating Hospital ship
Courtesy of Digital Collections and Archives, Tufts University.

Page vi: Child in life preserver
Courtesy of Digital Collections and Archives, Tufts University.

Pages viii ad ix: Map of Boston Harbor, 1884, S. Augustus Mitchell
Courtesy of Norman B. Leventhal Map Center, Boston Public Library.

Pages 2 and 3: Boston's Copley Square
Courtesy of the Library of Congress.

Page 4: Unity Street in Boston's North End.
Courtesy of the Library of Congress.

Page 5: Winter Street in Boston
Courtesy of the Trustees of the Boston Public Library.

Pages 12 and 13: Mothers and babies boarding ship
Courtesy of Digital Collections and Archives, Tufts University.

Page 14: Kindergarten Class
Courtesy of Digital Collections and Archives, Tufts University.

Page 16: Reverend Rufus Tobey
Courtesy of Tufts Medical Center.

Page 16: The Dover Street Bridge
Courtesy of the Boston Athenæum.

Page 17: Ten Time One Society Letter
Courtesy of Digital Collections and Archives, Tufts University.

Page 19: The Clifford and tugboat
Courtesy of Tufts Medical Center.

Page 20: Drawing of early days
Courtesy of Digital Collections and Archives, Tufts University.

Page 21: Newspaper headlines and drawings
Courtesy of Digital Collections and Archives, Tufts University.

Page 22: Embarking on the Clifford
Courtesy of Digital Collections and Archives, Tufts University.

Page 24: "Charity Money" and "No Benefit"
Courtesy of Digital Collections and Archives, Tufts University.

Page 25: "A Fine Entertainment"
Courtesy of Digital Collections and Archives, Tufts University.

Page 26: "Thou art so near and yet so far" drawing
Courtesy of Digital Collections and Archives, Tufts University.

Page 65: Mother with pram
Courtesy of the Library of Congress.

Pages 66 and 67: Shuttle car
Courtesy of Digital Collections and Archives, Tufts University.

Page 68: Ultraviolet treatment
Courtesy of Digital Collections and Archives, Tufts University.

Page 75: Metabolism crib
Courtesy of Digital Collections and Archives, Tufts University.

Page 77: Metabolism crib
Courtesy of Digital Collections and Archives, Tufts University.

Page 81: X-ray treatment
Courtesy of Digital Collections and Archives, Tufts University.

Page 82: Diathermy treatment
Courtesy of Digital Collections and Archives, Tufts University.

Page 84: Rickets treatment
Courtesy of Digital Collections and Archives, Tufts University.

Page 85: Hydrotherapy treatment
Courtesy of Digital Collections and Archives, Tufts University.

Page 86: Polio patient
Courtesy of Digital Collections and Archives, Tufts University.

Page 88: Humidified crib
Courtesy of Digital Collections and Archives, Tufts University.

Page 90 and 91: Student nurses
Courtesy of Digital Collections and Archives, Tufts University.

Page 92: Nurses in rowboat
Courtesy of Digital Collections and Archives, Tufts University.

Page 95: Premature jacket
Courtesy of Digital Collections and Archives, Tufts University.

Page 95: Breck feeder
Courtesy of Dr. John Kulig.

Page 101: Nurse tending to patients
Courtesy of Tufts Medical Center.

Pages 102 and 103: Nurses tending to patients
Courtesy of Digital Collections and Archives, Tufts University.

Pages 104 and 105: Open-air deck kindergarten class
Courtesy of Digital Collections and Archives, Tufts University.

Page 106: Open-air deck ward
Courtesy of Digital Collections and Archives, Tufts University.

Page 108: "Hurricane deck"
Courtesy of Digital Collections and Archives, Tufts University.

Page 111: North End Pier
Courtesy of Digital Collections and Archives, Tufts University.

Pages 116 and 117: Jackson Building playroom
Courtesy of Digital Collections and Archives, Tufts University.

Page 118: Mealtime on the open-air deck
Courtesy of Digital Collections and Archives, Tufts University.

Page 121: Jackson Building playroom
Courtesy of Digital Collections and Archives, Tufts University.

Page 122: Fresh air at the Jackson Building
Courtesy of Digital Collections and Archives, Tufts University.

Page 128: Miss Geneva Katz
Courtesy of Digital Collections and Archives, Tufts University.

Pages 130 and 131: Architectural design
Courtesy of Digital Collections and Archives, Tufts University.

Page 132: Jackson Building door
Courtesy of Digital Collections and Archives, Tufts University.

Page 135: Outside the On-Shore Department
Courtesy of Tufts Medical Center.

Page 138: Construction of new building
Courtesy of Digital Collections and Archives, Tufts University.

Page 141: Dr. Kreidberg and Ms. Katz
Courtesy of Digital Collections and Archives, Tufts University.

Page 142: Dr. Gellis
Courtesy of Digital Collections and Archives, Tufts University.

Pages 150 and 151:

Dr. Bowditch: *Courtesy of Countway Library, Harvard Medical School.*

Dr. Barron: *Courtesy of Digital Collections and Archives, Tufts University.*

Dr. Baty: *Courtesy of Tufts Medical Center.*

Dr. Kreidberg: *Courtesy of Tufts Medical Center.*

Dr. Gellis: *Courtesy of Digital Collections and Archives, Tufts University.*

Dr. Schaller: *Courtesy of Digital Collections and Archives, Tufts University.*

Dr. Franz: *Courtesy of Tufts Medical Center.*

Dr. Schreiber: *Courtesy of Tufts Medical Center.*

Pages 152 and 153: Linen room
Courtesy of Digital Collections and Archives, Tufts University.

Pages 148 and 149: Exterior of hospital
Courtesy of Tufts Medical Center.

Page 150: Dr. Radano
Courtesy of Tufts Medical Center.

Page 153: Dr. Sadeghi-Nejad
Courtesy of Tufts Medical Center.

Page 178: The Boston Floating Hospital ship
passing Boston Light
*Courtesy of Digital Collections and Archives,
Tufts University.*

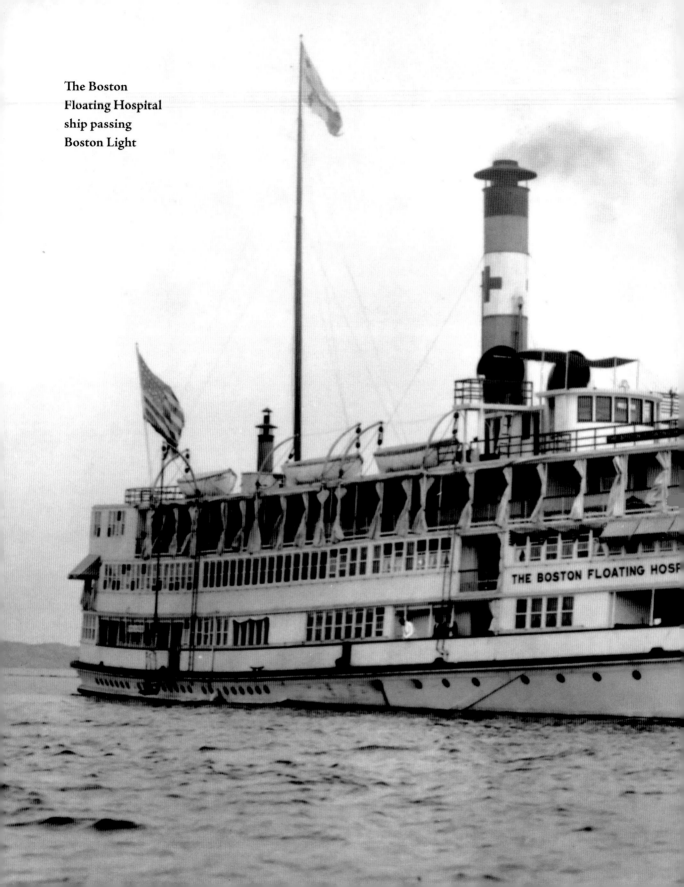

The Boston
Floating Hospital
ship passing
Boston Light

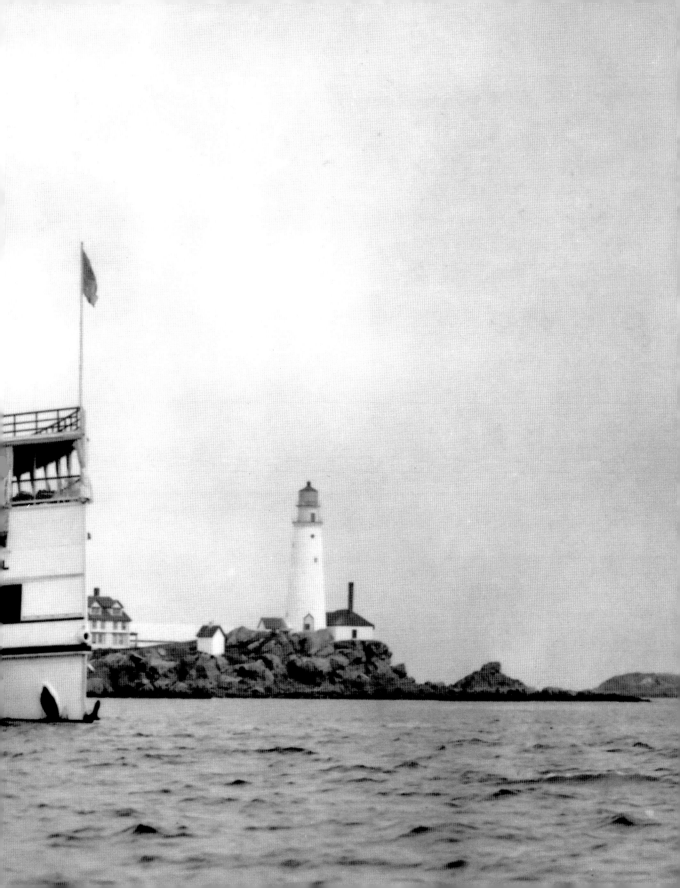